Renal Diet Cookbook For Beginners:

Help Yourself and your Loved Ones to Start a New Lifestyle. Enjoy the Benefits of Kidney-Friendly Food with Low-Sodium and Low-Potassium Easy and Tasty Recipes.

Olivia Braude

© Copyright 2022 by Olivia Braude - All rights reserved.

This document is geared towards providing exact and reliable information in regard to the topic and issue covered.

- From a Declaration of Principles which was accepted and approved equally by a Committee of the American Bar Association and a Committee of Publishers and Associations.

In no way is it legal to reproduce, duplicate, or transmit any part of this document in either electronic means or in printed format. All rights reserved.

The information provided herein is stated to be truthful and consistent, in that any liability, in terms of inattention or otherwise, by any usage or abuse of any policies, processes, or directions contained within is the solitary and utter responsibility of the recipient reader. Under no circumstances will any legal responsibility or blame be held against the publisher for any reparation, damages, or monetary loss due to the information herein, either directly or indirectly.

Respective authors own all copyrights not held by the publisher.

The information herein is offered for informational purposes solely and is universal as so. The presentation of the information is without contract or any type of guarantee assurance.

The trademarks that are used are without any consent, and the publication of the trademark is without permission or backing by the trademark owner. All trademarks and brands within this book are for clarifying purposes only and are owned by the owners themselves, not affiliated with this document.

Table of Contents

INTRODUCTION 8

What Is CKD: Symptoms, Risk Factors, Causes, Stage 10

    Chronic Kidney Disease (CKD) 11

    Causes of Kidney Disease 12

    Understanding the Symptoms 13

    The Five Stages of Kidney Disease 14

The Impact of Food on Your Kidneys 16

What Nutrients Do I Need to Regulate: Sodium, Potassium, Phosphorous, Protein, Fluids, Water? 18

Explanation of Diet Keywords 19

Tips For Living Well With CKD 22

Food To Avoid 27

Kidney-Friendly Food 33

Grocery List 35

    PHOSPHORUS TAB 37

    POTASSIUM TAB 39

Breakfast 41

1. Fast Microwave Egg Scramble 41
2. Raspberry Overnight Porridge 41
3. Summer Veggie Omelet 41
4. Yogurt Parfait with Strawberries 42
5. Apple and Onion Omelet 42
6. Apple Cherry Breakfast Risotto 43
7. Breakfast Burrito 43
8. Mushroom and Red Pepper Omelet 44
9. Mexican Scrambled Eggs in Tortilla 44
10. Mexican Style Burritos 45
11. Buckwheat and Grapefruit Porridge 45
12. Vegetable Omelet 46
13. Feta Mint Omelet 46
14. Pumpkin Apple Muffins 47
15. Feta And Bell Pepper Quiche 47
16. Quinoa Porridge 48
17. Egg and Veggie Muffins 48
18. Berry Chia with Yogurt 49
19. Arugula Eggs with Chili Peppers 49
20. Eggplant Chicken Sandwich 49
21. Grandma's Pancake Special 50

Salads 51

22. Thai Cucumber Salad 51
23. Butterscotch Apple Salad 51
24. Grapes Jicama Salad 51
25. Pineapple Berry Salad 52
26. Carrot Jicama Salad 52
27. Balsamic Beet Salad 52
28. Carrot Zucchini Salad 53
29. Broccoli Lettuce Salad 53
30. Farmer's Salad 53
31. Cucumber Salad 54
32. Barb's Asian Slaw 54

Condiments & Seasoning 55

33. Basil Pesto 55
34. Sweet Barbecue Sauce 55
35. Low-Sodium Mayonnaise 56

36.	Citrus and Mustard Marinade	56
37.	Fiery Honey Vinaigrette	56
38.	Buttermilk Herb Dressing	57
39.	Poppy Seed Dressing	57
40.	Mediterranean Dressing	57
41.	Fajita Rub	58
42.	Dried Herb Rub	58
43.	Mediterranean Seasoning	58
44.	Hot Curry Powder	59
45.	Cajun Seasoning	59
46.	Apple Pie Spice	60
47.	Ras El Hanout	60
48.	Poultry Seasoning	60
49.	Berbere Spice Mix	61

Snack and Appetizer 62

50.	Easy No-Bake Coconut Cookies	62
51.	Roasted Chili-Vinegar Peanuts	62
52.	Veggie Snack	62
53.	Healthy Spiced Nuts	63
54.	Roasted Asparagus	63
55.	Low-Fat Mango Salsa	63
56.	Carrot and Parsnips French Fries	64
57.	Apple & Strawberry Snack	64
58.	Candied Macadamia Nuts	64
59.	Baba Ghanouj	65
60.	Herbal Cream Cheese Tartines	65
61.	Spicy Crab Dip	66
62.	Blueberry-Ricotta Swirl	66
63.	Cranberry Cabbage	67

64.	Carrot-Apple Casserole	67
65.	Garlic Mashed Potatoes	67

Soups & Stews 69

66.	Chicken Noodle Soup	69
67.	Classic Chicken Soup	69
68.	Beef Okra Soup	70
69.	Chicken Pasta Soup	70
70.	Cabbage Turkey Soup	71
71.	Chicken Fajita Soup	71
72.	Cream of Chicken Soup	72
73.	Turkey & Lemon-Grass Soup	72
74.	Paprika Pork Soup	73
75.	White Fish Stew	73
76.	Pumpkin, Coconut and Sage Soup	73
77.	The Kale and Green Lettuce Soup	74
78.	Sweet Potato and Corn Soup	74
79.	Chickpea Curry Soup	75
80.	Onion, Kale and White Bean Soup	75

Meat & Poultry 77

81.	Creamy Chicken	77
82.	Grilled Chicken Pizza	77
83.	Lemon & Herb Chicken Wraps	77
84.	Cherry Chicken Salad	78
85.	Southern Fried Chicken	78
86.	Carrot & Ginger Chicken Noodles	79
87.	Cilantro Drumsticks	79
88.	Chicken Sauté	80
89.	Rosemary Chicken	80

#	Recipe	Page
90.	Chicken Strawberry Green Lettuce Salad with Ginger-Lime Dressing	81
91.	Creamy Turkey	81
92.	Parmesan And Basil Turkey Salad	82
93.	Oven-Baked Turkey Thighs	82
94.	Turkey Sausages	83
95.	Pork with Bell Pepper	83
96.	Pork Loins with Leeks	84
97.	Chinese Beef Wraps	84
98.	Beef Ragu	84
99.	Country Fried Steak	85
100.	Beef Pot Roast	85
101.	Homemade Burgers	86
102.	Roast Beef	86
103.	Ginger & Bean Sprout Steak Stir-Fry	87
104.	Beef Brochettes	87
105.	Lamb with Prunes	88
106.	Spiced Lamb Burgers	88
107.	Lamb with Zucchini & Couscous	89

Seafood **90**

#	Recipe	Page
108.	Shrimp Paella	90
109.	Salmon & Pesto Salad	90
110.	Baked Fennel & Garlic Sea Bass	91
111.	4-Ingredients Salmon Fillet	91
112.	Spanish Cod in Sauce	92
113.	Haddock & Buttered Leeks	92
114.	Thai Spiced Halibut	92
115.	Monkfish Curry	93
116.	Tuna Noodle Casserole	93
117.	Citrus Tuna Ceviche	94
118.	Cilantro and Chili Infused Swordfish	94
119.	Cooked Tilapia with Mango Salsa	95
120.	Herb-Crusted Baked Haddock	95
121.	Baked Cod with Salsa	96
122.	Cilantro-Lime Flounder	96
123.	Halibut with Lemon Caper Sauce	97
124.	Jambalaya	97
125.	Shrimp Szechuan	98
126.	Baked Fish à la Mushrooms	98
127.	Shrimp and Asparagus Linguine	99
128.	Old Fashioned Salmon Soup	99
129.	Lemony Haddock	100
130.	Glazed Salmon	100
131.	Tuna Casserole	101
132.	Oregano Salmon with Crunchy Crust	101
133.	Sardine Fish Cakes	101
134.	Cajun Catfish	102
135.	Poached Gennaro/Seabass with Red Peppers	102
136.	Oregano Grilled Calamari	103
137.	Nice Coconut Haddock	103

Side Dishes **104**

#	Recipe	Page
138.	Cauliflower and Leeks	104
139.	Eggplant and Mushroom Sauté	104
140.	Mint Zucchini	104
141.	Celery and Kale Mix	105
142.	Kale, Mushrooms and Red Chard Mix	105
143.	Bok Choy and Beets	106
144.	Broccoli and Almonds Mix	106

145.	Squash and Cranberries 106	172.	Baked Eggplants Slices 119
146.	Creamy Chard 107	173.	Fast Cabbage Cakes 120
147.	Dill Carrots 107	174.	Cilantro Chili Burgers 120
148.	Thai-Style Eggplant Dip 108		

Smoothies & Drinks 122

149.	Collard Salad Rolls with Peanut Dipping Sauce 108	175.	Very Berry Smoothie 122
		176.	Raspberry Peach Breakfast Smoothie 122
150.	Simple Roasted Broccoli 109	177.	Mango Lassi Smoothie 122
151.	Roasted Mint Carrots 109	178.	Breakfast Smoothie 123
152.	Roasted Root Vegetables 110	179.	Apple And Beet Juice Mix 123
153.	Vegetable Couscous 110	180.	Assorted Fresh Fruit Juice 123
154.	Ginger Cauliflower Rice 111	181.	Berry Mint Water 124
155.	Basil Zucchini Spaghetti 111	182.	Fennel Digestive Cooler 124
156.	Braised Cabbage 112	183.	Tropical Juice 124
		184.	Green Tea with Arugula Leaves, Lime, And Kale Leaves... 124

Vegetarian & Vegan 113

157.	Mixed Pepper Paella 113		
158.	Minted Zucchini Noodles 113	185.	Winter Berry Milkshake 125
159.	Vegan Alfredo Fettuccine Pasta 114	186.	Pineapple Juice 125

Desserts 126

160.	Chinese Tempeh Stir Fry 114		
161.	Pesto Pasta Salad 115	187.	Pudding Glass with Banana and Whipped Cream 126
162.	Asparagus Fried Rice 115		
163.	Vegetarian Taco Salad 116	188.	Pumpkin Cheesecake 126
164.	Sautéed Green Beans 116	189.	Small Chocolate Cakes 127
165.	Garlicky Penne Pasta with Asparagus 117	190.	Amarena Dessert 127
166.	Garlic Mashed Carrots 117	191.	Strawberry Ice Cream 127
167.	Double-Boiled Country Style Fried Carrots 117	192.	Grilled Peach Sundaes 128
168.	Broccoli-Onion Latkes 118	193.	Almond Butter Mousse 128
169.	Glazed Snap Peas 118	194.	Keto Panna Cotta 128
170.	Steamed Collard Greens 119	195.	Spiced Peaches 129
171.	Cauliflower Rice 119	196.	Pumpkin Cheesecake Bar 129
		197.	Blueberry Mini Muffins 130

198.	*Lemon Mousse........................ 130*	*WEEK 1 .... 133*
199.	*Raspberry Popsicle................. 131*	*WEEK 2 .... 134*
200.	*Coconut Loaf.......................... 131*	*WEEK 3 .... 135*
201.	*Dessert Cocktail 132*	*WEEK 4 .... 136*
202.	*Baked Egg Custard 132*	**Conclusion 137**

Meal Plans 133

INTRODUCTION

To maintain a safe and healthy diet, it is important to be aware of dietary needs. It's always a good idea for those who have specific dietary needs to consult with a doctor, dietician, or nutritionist. This book will go over some basic information about Renal Diet as well as just how to maintain one.

The Renal Diet is designed to help people with kidney problems. It restricts the amount of protein and salt in a person's diet.

As many as 1 in 3 adults age 20 and older has chronic kidney disease (CKD). And unfortunately, this number is steadily increasing as we grow older. One of the most serious complications of CKD is high blood pressure, which may lead to further health complications such as heart attack or stroke. People with CKD are also at risk for life-threatening conditions such as anemia, especially those on dialysis treatments.

The first step before starting a renal diet is understanding that kidneys are an organ that filters waste from the blood and removes it from the body through urine. When kidneys become damaged or diseased, they can no longer handle this job adequately. A lot of the filtering and removal of waste is done by the liver. When this function has been compromised, a person can experience some serious symptoms, such as jaundice, which is characterized by yellow skin and eyes.

The kidneys are located on either side of your spine and are attached to it via a large blood supply. This blood supply is called the renin-angiotensin system. When this system becomes damaged, it can cause problems in various other systems of your body, including heart and even the immune system.

The Renal Diet was originally developed by a group of urologists and nutritionists in order to help people with kidney problems avoid these issues. The diet is designed to help control blood pressure and reduce the protein levels in the body, both of which can help slow down the progression of CKD.

A major component of the Renal Diet is getting fluid intake under control. The National Kidney Foundation encourages everyone to drink plenty of water every day, but for those on a Renal Diet, this is even more important. Drinking enough water will help flush out sodium by transporting it out through urination.

In addition, the Renal Diet limits the amount of protein that a person is allowed to consume. Evidence shows that high levels of protein in the body can increase blood pressure. In order to keep protein levels under control, a limit of 0.6 grams per kilogram of body weight is recommended.

One important part of the Renal Diet is to not rely on products that are high in sodium or sugar. When you're on a Renal Diet, it's generally a good idea to limit your sodium intake to 2,000 milligrams per day. This amount can be found in about 2 teaspoons of salt or 1/4 cup of table salt. Sugar should also be limited to no more than 25 grams per day.

The following are some tips and tricks to help you get started on the Renal Diet:

- Start gradually. The National Kidney Foundation recommends starting your Renal Diet slow by cutting down on sodium intake and slowly incorporating more foods from the "yes" list. If you need to, cut back on sodium by using less table salt and eating fewer processed foods.

- Protein can be found in many different sources, including meats, fish, poultry and tofu. Most of these foods are also high in fat, so it's recommended that you make small adjustments to your diet over time to avoid drastically cutting out fat.

- The Renal Diet is designed for adults with CKD stage 3 or higher. If you have been diagnosed with stage 3 CKD or above, you should follow the dietary guidelines as closely as possible.

- If you haven't been diagnosed with CKD but your doctor thinks that you may be at risk of developing it, you should still try to follow the guidelines as closely as possible.

Always consult with your doctor before starting any new diet or changing your old one.

What Is CKD: Symptoms, Risk Factors, Causes, Stages

It is said that 10% of life is what happens to you, while the remaining 90% comprises your reactions to the things that happen to you. There is a considerable degree of truth to that. When you think about it, the things that are beyond our control cannot be influenced by us. So why do we yearn to control them? Why do we exert so much effort, time, and attention to change the direction of the immovable forces in our life? Why do we stubbornly force ourselves to face more disappointments when the same energy that we force into the uncontrollable factors in our life can yield spectacular results in the controllable or manageable areas of our lives?

We're doing this because we're worried about the consequences of losing control. We imagine that things might spiral out of control to a point where they are going to become truly calamitous. Another version of this thought process is where we do not like it when things take a course in our lives that we are not comfortable with. When it comes to things we cannot control, they might create a favorable scenario or cause disasters. That is not a risk we would like to take. Yet, despite knowing that our actions to influence the situation is futile, we try anyway, hoping that perhaps—through some divine intervention or miracle—something will happen.

Kidney function or renal functions are the terms used to explain how well kidneys work. A healthy individual is born with a pair of kidneys. This is why whenever one of the kidneys lost its function, it went unnoticed due to the function of the other kidney. But if the kidney functions further drop altogether and reach a level as low as 25 percent, it turns out to be serious for the patients. People who only have one kidney-functioning need proper external therapy and, in worst cases, a kidney transplant.

Kidney diseases occur when a number of renal cells known as nephrons are partially or completely damaged and do not properly filter incoming blood. The gradual damage to the kidney cells can occur due to various reasons, sometimes it is the acidic or toxic build-up inside the kidney over time, other times it is genetic, or the result of other kidney damaging diseases like hypertension (high blood pressure) or diabetes.

1. Chronic Kidney Disease (CKD)

CKD or Chronic Kidney Disease is the stage of kidney damage where it fails to filter the blood properly. The term chronic is used to refer to gradual and long-term damage to an organ. Chronic kidney disease is therefore developed after slow yet progressive damage to the kidneys. The symptoms of this disease only appear when the toxic wastes start to build up in the body. Therefore, such a stage should be prevented at all costs. Hence, early diagnosis of the disease proves to be significant. The sooner the patient realizes the gravity of the situation, the better measures he can take to curb the problem.

What about after we are affected by diseases? Well, even then, we make sure that we spend less time pondering about and trying to change what we cannot do and more time on how to take care of ourselves. By focusing on our own actions, we gain more confidence, motivation, and knowledge. We realize that the ability to make changes, however big or small, lies within us.

In the case of chronic kidney disease, we have the ability to prevent the condition from progressing.

2. Causes of Kidney Disease

According to the National Kidney Foundation, the two main causes of chronic kidney disease are high blood pressure and diabetes (National Kidney Foundation, n.d.). If you visit a doctor, health expert, or diet consultant, then you will realize that one of the major ways to manage your blood pressure and prevent diabetes is a healthy diet.

As the blood pressure or diabetes levels get worse, so does the amount of waste build-up. The waste goes into your blood faster and kidneys have to filter them. At this point, your kidneys are like an overworked employee at a firm; there is so much work remaining, but only a small amount of time to get finished during a particular period. Kidneys start to deteriorate over time. The filters begin to leak, unable to hold on to the waste build-up anymore. Only a small percentage of the entire waste gets filtered properly, with the rest entering the bloodstream. For some, the time it takes for kidney failure might be months, while for others, the kidneys could worsen across a span of years. It all depends on numerous factors like diet, lifestyle choices, and even genetics.

Pretty soon, you might feel like your kidney functions have been kidnapped; they don't seem to be working well anymore or they barely exist. Think of the example of the overworked employee that we used earlier. At some point, the employee could collapse out of dehydration or exhaustion. In a similar way, the kidney disease causes the organs to fail, which causes numerous problems such as low energy, high exhaustion levels, sleep difficulties, poor appetite, swollen ankles and feet, and the need to urinate more often, especially at night.

3. Understanding the Symptoms

The good thing is that we can prevent the chronic stage of renal disease by identifying the early signs of any form of kidney damage. Even when a person feels minor changes in his body, he should consult an expert to confirm if it might lead to something serious. The following are a few of the early symptoms of renal damage:

- Tiredness or drowsiness
- Muscle cramps
- Loss of appetite
- Changes in the frequency of urination
- Swelling of hands and feet
- A feeling of itchiness
- Numbness
- The darkness of skin
- Trouble in sleeping
- Shortness of breath
- The feeling of nausea or vomiting

These symptoms can appear in combination with one another. These are general signs of body malfunction, and they should never be ignored. And if they are left unnoticed, they can lead to worsening of the condition and may appear as:

- Back pain
- Abdominal pain
- Fever
- Rash
- Diarrhea
- Nosebleeds
- Vomiting

After witnessing any of these symptoms, a person should immediately consult a health expert and prepare himself or herself for the required lifestyle changes.

4. The Five Stages of Kidney Disease

Chronic kidney disease is categorized into five stages, each one characterized by a certain degree of damage done to the kidneys and rate of glomerular filtration, which is the rate at which filtration takes place in the kidneys. These help us understand just how well the kidneys are functioning.

Stage 1

The first stage is the least severe and actually comes close to a healthy state of your kidneys. Most people will never be aware if they have entered stage 1 of chronic kidney disease or CKD. In many cases, if people discover stage 1 CKD, then it is because they were being tested for diabetes or high blood pressure. Otherwise, people can find out about stage 1 CKD if they discover protein or blood in the urine, signs of kidney damage in an ultrasound, a computerized tomography (CT) scan, or through magnetic resonance imaging (MRI). If people have a family history of polycystic kidney disease (PKD), then there are chances that they might have CKD as well.

Stage 2

In this stage, there is a mild decrease in the glomerular filtration rate. People don't usually notice any symptoms at this stage as well. The reasons for discovering any signs of CKD are the same as the reasons provided in stage 1.

So, what's the difference between stage 1 and stage 2? It all lies in the glomerular filtration rate, or GFR for short. The GFR is measured in milliliters/minute.

In stage 1, the glomerular filtration rate (GFR) is around 90 ml/min. The normal range of the GFR is from 90 ml/min to 120 ml/min. So, as you can see, stage 1 CKD shows a GFR at the lower end of the range. Because it falls so close to a normal rate, it easily goes unnoticed. At stage 2, the GFR falls to between 60-89 ml/min. You might become concerned with the range stage 2 falls in, but your kidneys are actually resilient. Even if they are not functioning at 100 percent, your kidneys are capable of doing a good job. So good that you might not notice anything was out of the ordinary.

Even though the differences between stage 1 and 2 are minuscule, they cannot be combined because the chances of someone showing certain symptoms of CKD when in stage 2 are greater.

Stage 3

At this stage, the kidneys suffer moderate damage. In order to properly gauge the level of damage, this stage is further divided into two: stage 3A and stage 3B. The reason for the division is that even though the severity of the disease worsens from 3A to 3B, the damage to the kidneys is still within moderate levels.

Each of the divisions is characterized by their GFR.

- 3A has a GFR between 45–59 ml/min.
- 3B has a GFR between 30–44 ml/min.

When patients reach stage 3, they begin to experience other symptoms of CKD, which include the below:

- Increase in fatigue.
- Shortness of breath and swelling of extremities also called edema.
- Slight kidney pain, where the pain is felt in the lower back area.
- Change in the color of urine.

Stage 4

At stage 4, the kidney disease becomes severe. The GFR falls down to 15–30 ml/min. As the waste build-up increases, the patient might experience nausea and vomiting, a build-up of urea in the blood that could cause bad breath, and find themselves having trouble doing everyday tasks such as reading a newspaper or trying to write up an email.

When a patient reaches stage 4, it is critical to contact a nephrologist (a doctor who specializes in renal disorders).

Stage 5

At stage 5, the kidneys have a GFR of less than 15 ml/min. This is a truly low rate that causes the build-up of waste to reach a critical point. The organs have reached an advanced stage of CKD, causing them to lose almost all their abilities in order to function normally.

The Impact of Food on Your Kidneys

The kidneys have a delicate balancing act to perform. They need to keep the body's levels of substances that are toxic, such as potassium, sodium and phosphorus in balance at all times. In addition, they also need to filter blood and maintain a balance between too much fluid on one side of the body, or too little fluid on the other side. Excess fluids can lead to congestion from an area of the body where there are not enough fluids - a condition called peripheral oedema. This can be seen in the legs when standing or in the face as swelling under the eyes.

The kidney's function is controlled by a hormone called erythropoietin (EPO), produced by the kidneys. EPO is released into the circulatory system to stimulate red blood cell production, thereby ensuring that there is enough oxygen taken around the body by these cells. EPO is also important to bone health as it stimulates bone marrow to produce cells that give rise to all three types of blood cell found in blood: red cells, white cells and platelets.

Eating **sodium** rich foods or drinks will mean that too much fluid is retained within the body and can result in fluid collection around the ankles (peripheral oedema) or face. The kidneys may also be damaged with long term exposure to high sodium levels.

Potassium is a mineral found in most food. Potassium rich foods are those rich in fruits and vegetables, legumes, nuts and seeds. Potassium plays an important role in blood pressure control and the contraction of muscles, including the heart muscle.

Phosphorus is one of the main building blocks of bones and teeth. It is needed in smaller amounts than calcium and vitamin C during childhood and adolescence, however adult bones need slightly more phosphorus. These days there is a lot dietary phosphorus in our food, most commonly from soft drinks and processed foods such as burgers, junk food like crisps or fast-food meals containing chicken nuggets - which are often deep fried in oil with added salt.

Excess phosphorus can lead to problems for your kidneys as it takes them away from their role as waste managers within your body. Your kidneys will then not be able to filter the blood effectively and excess minerals such as phosphorus, potassium and calcium may build up in your circulation which can lead to other issues.

These issues include a condition called renal osteodystrophy. This is where excessive amounts of calcium may lead to excessive hardening of the bones in both children and adults. It causes pain in the back, legs and hips which get worse over time without treatment. The disease is most common world-wide in African-Americans, Native Americans and Asian Indians but can be seen occasionally in people of European descent as well.

Vitamin D3 is important for maintaining good kidney health. Some people may think they don't need vitamin D but it is actually quite important, which is why it is wise to ensure you are getting adequate amounts from food sources such as fatty fish and eggs, given that vitamin D from sunlight tends not be as effective.

Probiotics are live micro-organisms which when administered in adequate amounts help to maintain the health of the intestinal tract. These have been shown to be particularly beneficial for dialysis patients, helping their immune systems and potentially their kidneys.

The ideal diet can be summarized in four words – reduce your phosphorus intake wherever possible and eat more potassium rich foods such as fruits, vegetables, legumes and nuts/seeds.

What Nutrients Do I Need to Regulate: Sodium, Potassium, Phosphorous, Protein, Fluids, Water?

If you have been diagnosed with kidney dysfunction, a proper diet is necessary for controlling the amount of toxic waste in the bloodstream. When toxic waste piles up in the system along with increased fluid, chronic inflammation occurs, and we have a much higher chance of developing cardiovascular, bone, metabolic, or other health issues.

Renal Diet improve the quality of life for patients with renal disease.

Your doctor can give you more advice than this, and you should always let him or her know if your situation improves.

If you choose to use a dietitian, they can point you precisely to what you should and shouldn't consume and why. Being aware of the effect food has on your body is important and can help you feel good every day. Also, this design is not an alternative to clinical guidelines. Yet Renal Diet help most kidney disease sufferers to become and stay healthier.

Since your kidneys can't fully get rid of the waste on their own, which comes from food and drinks, probably the only natural way to help our system is through this diet.

A Renal Diet is especially useful during the first stages of kidney dysfunction and leads to the following benefits:

- Prevents excess fluid and waste build-up.

- Prevents the progression of renal dysfunction stages.

- Decreases the likelihood of developing other chronic health problems, e.g., heart disorders

- It has a mild antioxidant function in the body, which keeps inflammation and inflammatory responses under control.

The above-mentioned benefits are noticeable once the patient follows the diet for at least a month and then continues it for longer periods to avoid the stage where dialysis is needed.

The strictness of the diet is determined by the present stage of renal/kidney disease; if you are in the third or fourth stage, for example, you should adhere to a tighter diet and pay close attention to the foods that are permitted or prohibited.

These exact foods and nutrients that you should take when following a renal diet will be given to you in the following sections, so keep reading.

Explanation of Diet Keywords

The following nutrients are important in a renal diet since some can help improve the condition while others can aggravate it. Essentially, the renal diet is based on low consumption of certain nutrients like potassium and phosphorus simply because it promotes fluid build-up within the system of a CKD patient. Here is a brief explanation of the function of each nutrient and its role in a renal diet:

Potassium

Potassium is a mineral that naturally occurs in certain foods and plays a role in regulating heart rhythm and muscle movement. It is also needed for keeping fluid and electrolyte balance at normal levels. Our kidneys keep only the right levels of potassium in our system, and when it is excess, they expel it via the urine.

The problem is that once kidneys can't function properly, all this excess potassium can't be expelled out and spikes up, causing symptoms like muscle and bone weakness, abnormal heartbeat, and heart failure in extreme cases.

A diet low in potassium is recommended to prevent build-up and avoid such negative side effects.

Sodium

Sodium is a trace mineral that is found in most foods that we eat today and it is the key component of salt, which is actually a sodium compound mixed with chloride. Most food that we consume and especially processed food are highly loaded with salt; however, we may be eating sodium in other forms, too, e.g., fish. The key role of sodium is to regulate blood pressure, regulate nerve function, and maintain the balance of acids in the blood. However, when sodium is excessively high and the kidneys cannot expel it, it can lead to the following symptoms: an elevated feeling of thirst, swelling of hands, feet and the face, elevated blood pressure, and problems with breathing.

This is why it is suggested to keep sodium intake low to avoid the above.

Phosphorus

Phosphorus is an essential mineral that is responsible for the development and regeneration of our bones. Phosphorus also plays a key role in the growth of connective tissue, e.g., muscles and the regulation of muscle motions. When the food we eat contains phosphorus, it gets absorbed by the intestines and then gets deposited in our bones.

However, when kidneys are damaged or dysfunctioning, the excess phosphorus can't be expelled through our systems and causes problems such as: extracting calcium out of the bones/making them weaker, and leading to excess calcium in the bloodstream that interferes with blood vessels, heart, eye, and lung function.

Protein

Protein is a nutritional compound that consists of amino acids, which play a key role in various system functions like cell communication, oxygen supply, and cellular metabolism. They are also a part of a healthy immune system.

Normally, protein is not an issue for our kidneys. When protein is metabolized, waste by-products are also created and are filtered through the kidneys. This waste, along with extrarenal proteins after will be expelled through urine.

However, when kidneys are unable to filter out excess protein, it gets accumulated in the blood and cause problems.

This doesn't mean that renal disease patients should avoid protein totally as it is still necessary for some metabolic functions, as long as it's taken in moderate amounts and based on the stage of renal disease.

Carbs

Carbs act as a key source of fuel for our bodies. The consumption of carbs is turned into glucose in our system, which is a primary source of energy.

Carbs are ok to be eaten in moderation by kidney patients and the daily recommended allowance is up to 150 grams/day. However, patients that also have diabetes (besides renal disease) should control their carb consumption to avoid any sudden spikes in their blood glucose.

Fats

Being in balanced amounts, fats in our bodies act as an energy source, aid in the release of hormones, and regulate blood pressure. They also carry some vitamins that are fat-soluble such as A, D, E, and K, which are also very important for our systems. However, not all fats are created alike; some are beneficial to our health while others are detrimental. Bad fats are saturated and trans fats are found in processed meat, dairy, and other products. They are also found in margarine and vegetable fat shortenings.

In general, fats don't pose a risk for renal disease patients; however, it is suggested to limit the consumption of saturated and trans fats to avoid any cardiovascular problems, e.g., elevated blood pressure and clogging of the arteries.

Dietary Fiber

Dietary fiber is a compound that can't be digested on its own by enzymes and acids in our stomach and intestines but is needed for the system to aid in the digestion of our food and encourage bowel movements. They generally promote bowel regularity and decrease the likelihood of developing constipation inside the colon. Dietary fiber is typically found in fruits, vegetables, seeds, and whole grains.

In patients with renal disease, dietary fiber is ok up to 28 grams/day as long as these plant foods don't contain high amounts of phosphorus or potassium.

Vitamins

According to medical and dietary guidelines, our bodies need close to 13 vitamins to function. Vitamins play a key role in metabolic functions and the normal functioning of our cardiovascular, digestive, nervous system, and immune systems. The adoption of a nutritionally dense and balanced diet is necessary for getting all the vitamins our system needs. However, due to some diet restrictions, e.g., sodium, many renal patients are in need of water-soluble vitamins like B-complex (B1, B2, B6, B12, folic acid, and biotin) and small amounts of Vitamin C.

Minerals

Minerals are needed for our system to maintain healthy connective tissue e.g., bones, muscles, and skin, and facilitate the normal function of our hearts and central nervous systems.

Our kidneys typically expel any excess amount of minerals through our urine, as some can lead to health symptoms, e.g., muscle spasms when their levels are abnormally high.

Some minerals like potassium and phosphorus cannot be expelled by our kidneys when in excess, and so their intake through diet should be limited.

Other trace minerals are perfectly fine when following a renal diet: iron, copper, zinc, and selenium. A lack of these can lead to increased oxidative stress so it is important to take sufficient amounts through diet or supplementation.

Fluids

Fluids are necessary for the proper hydration of our systems in fact, lack of fluids can lead to dehydration and death in extreme cases.

However, in patients with renal dysfunction, fluids can quickly build-up to the point of placing pressure on vital organs like the lungs and heart and becoming dangerous. This is the reason why many physicians advise their kidney patients to limit the consumption of fluids, especially during the last stages of the disorder.

Tips For Living Well With CKD

A kidney disease diagnosis can seem devastating at first. The news may come as a shock for some people, who may not have experienced any symptoms. It's important to remember that you can control your own progress and improvement through diet and lifestyle changes, even when a prognosis is serious. Taking steps to improve your health can make a significant effort to slow the progression of kidney disease and improve your quality of life.

Tip 1: Focus on Weight Loss Lose the Extra Weight

Losing weight is one of the most common reasons for going on a diet. It's also one of the most effective ways to treat and prevent kidney disease from worsening. Carrying excess weight contributes to high toxicity levels in the body by storing toxins instead of releasing them through the kidneys. Eating foods high in trans fats, sugar, and excess sodium contribute to obesity, which affects close to one-third of North Americans and continues to rise in many other countries where fast foods are becoming easier to access and less expensive. Losing weight is a difficult cycle for many who often diet temporarily only to return to unhealthy habits after reaching a milestone, which results in gaining the weight back, causing an unhealthy "yo-yo" diet effect.

There are some basic and easy changes you can make to shed those first pounds, which will begin to take the pressure off the kidneys and help you onto the path of regular weight loss:

• Drink plenty of water. If you can't drink eight glasses of water every day, try adding unsweetened natural sparkling water or herbal teas.

• Reduce the amount of sugar and carbohydrates you consume. This doesn't require adapting to a ketogenic or low-carb diet—you'll notice a major change after ditching soda and reducing the bread and pasta by half.

• Take your time to eat and avoid rushing. If you need to eat in a hurry, grab a piece of fruit or a small portion of macadamia nuts. Avoid sugary and salty foods as much as possible. Choose fresh fruits over potato chips and chocolate bars.

• Create a short-list of kidney-friendly foods that you enjoy and use this as your reference or guide when grocery shopping. This will help you stock up on snacks, ingredients, and foods for your kitchen that work well within your renal diet plan, at the same time reducing your chances of succumbing to the temptation of eating a bag of salted pretzels or chocolate.

Once you take a few steps towards changing the way you eat, it will get easier. Making small changes at first is the key to success and to progressing with a new way of eating and living. If you are already in the habit of consuming packaged foods—such as crackers, chips, processed dips, sauces, and sodas, for example—try cutting down on one or two items at a time, and over a period of time gradually eliminate and cut down other items. Slowly replace these with fresh foods and healthier choices, so that your body has a chance to adapt without extreme cravings that often occur during sudden changes.

Tip 2: Quit Smoking and Reduce Alcohol

It's not easy to quit smoking or using recreational drugs, especially when they have been used for a long time and the effects have already made an impact on your health. At some point, you'll begin to notice a difference in the way you feel and how your body changes over time. This includes chronic coughing related to respiratory conditions, shortness of breath, and a lack of energy.

For most people, quitting "cold turkey" or all at once is not an option because of the withdrawal symptoms and increased chances of starting again. However, this method can work if applied with a strong support system and a lot of determination, though it's not the best option for everyone. Reducing smoking on your own, or switching to e-cigarettes or a patch or medication, can help significantly over time. Setting goals of reduction until the point of quitting can be a beneficial way to visualize success and provide a sense of motivation. The following tips may also be useful for quitting smoking and other habit-forming substances:

Join a support group and talk to other people who relate to you. Share your struggles, ideas, and thoughts, which will help others as well as yourself during this process.

- Track your progress on a calendar or in a notebook, either by pen and paper or on an application. This can serve as a motivator and as a way to display how you've done so far and where you can improve. For example, you may have reduced your smoking from ten to seven cigarettes per day, then increased to nine. This may indicate a slight change that can be considered to focus on reducing your intake further, from nine cigarettes to seven or six per day, and so on.

- Be aware of stress factors in your life that cause you to smoke or use substances. If these factors are avoidable, make every effort to minimize or stop them from impacting your life. This may include specific people, places, or situations that can "trigger" a craving or make you feel more likely to use it than usual. If there are situations that you cannot avoid, such as family, work, or school-related situations, consult with a trusted friend or someone you can confide in who can be present with you during these instances.

- Don't be afraid to ask for help. Many people cannot quit on their own without at least some assistance from others. Seeking the guidance and expertise of a counselor or medical professional to better yourself can be one of the most important decisions you make to improve the quality of your life.

Alcoholic Beverages: To Quit or Reduce Consumption?

Alcoholic beverages are often enjoyed with a good meal or at a social event, and for some people, drinking outside of these circumstances or events is not frequent. For these people, moderately drinking alcohol is a lifestyle that doesn't have too much impact on their health and is not habit-forming. Drinking frequently and/or binge drinking can present a problem for many people and can have a detrimental effect on the kidneys. Heavy drinking can be the result of alcoholism, which often needs professional treatment or assistance, where the impact on your health becomes severe. For moderate to light drinkers, continuing to drink small amounts is acceptable during early to moderate stages of kidney disease, though it should be avoided completely if on dialysis. The key to reducing or quitting alcohol is not the same for everyone. Some people are prone to addictive traits, which include dependence on substances like alcohol. Unfortunately, it is a lifelong habit that can take a toll on a person's physical and mental well-being—through the right support and a healthy diet, it can be overcome.

There are some simple changes to make that can improve your chances of successfully reducing alcohol consumption, whether the aim is to quit completely or cut back on drinking—both of which are important goals to consider when working towards a healthier lifestyle:

•	When attending a social event, alternate between a beverage and a glass of water (or sparkling water). This will allow your body to absorb the alcohol before consuming too much, as well as allow you to flush the drink with water and cut down on your consumption.

•	Drink slowly and eat in between, even if just a snack. This will give your body a chance to digest and absorb more effectively and by slowing the pace of drinking you are reducing your chances of consuming too much at once.

•	Avoid keeping alcohol at home, if you feel that it will encourage more drinking rather than less. If you choose to buy alcohol, keep just enough to enjoy for special occasions and limit the amount you have at a time.

Tip 3: Getting Active Adding Movement and Exercise to Your Lifestyle

One of the most important ways to keep fit and healthy is by staying active and engaging in regular exercise. Regular movement is the key and exercise is different for everyone, depending on their abilities and available options. Fortunately, there are unlimited ways to customize an exercise routine or plan that can suit any lifestyle. For many people experiencing kidney disease, one of the major struggles is losing weight and living a sedentary life, where movement is minimal and exercise is not practiced. Smoking, eating processed foods, and not getting the required nutrition can further impact the body in such a way that exercise is seen as a hurdle and a challenge that is best avoided. Making lifestyle changes is not something that should be done all at once, but over a period of time—especially during the early stages of renal disease—so the impact of the condition is minimized over time and becomes more manageable.

Where can you begin, if you haven't exercised at all or for a long period of time? For starters, don't sign up for a marathon or engage in any strenuous activities unless it is safe to do so. Start slow, and take your time. Before taking on any new movements—whether it is minimal, low-impact walking or stretching, or a more moderate to the high-impact regimen—always talk to your doctor to rule out any impact this may have on other existing conditions, such as blood pressure and respiratory conditions, as well as your kidneys. Most, if not all, physicians will likely recommend exercise as part of the treatment plan, but may advise beginning slowly if your body isn't used to exercise.

Simple techniques to introduce exercise into your life require a commitment. This can begin with a quick 15-minute walk or jog and a 10-minute or 15-minute stretch in the morning before starting your day. Some easy and introductory techniques to consider are the following:

- Take a walk for 10 to 15 minutes each day, at least three or four days each week. If you find it difficult at first, due to cramping, respiratory issues, or other conditions, walk slowly and breathe deeply. Make sure you feel relaxed during your walks. Find a scenic path or area in your neighborhood that is pleasant and gives you something to enjoy, such as a beautiful sunset or forested park. Keep yourself hydrated by bringing a bottle of water.

- Stretch for five minutes once a day. This doesn't mean you need to do any intricate yoga poses or specific techniques. In fact, moving your ankles, wrists, and arms in circles and standing every so often (if you sit often) and twisting your torso can help release stress and improve your blood flow, which lowers blood pressure and helps your body transport nutrients to areas in need of repair.

- Practice breathing long, measured breaths. This will help prepare you for more endurance-based exercise, such as jogging, long walks, cycling, and swimming. Count to five on each inhale and exhale, and practice moving slowly as you breathe, to "sync" or coordinate your body's movements with your breathing. If you have difficulty with the respiratory system, take it slow and don't push yourself. Stop immediately if you feel weak or out of breath and try again later or the next day at a slower speed.

- Start a beginner's yoga class and learn the fundamentals of various poses and stretches. It is helpful to arrive early and speak with the instructor, who can provide guidance on which modifications work best, if needed. They may also be able to provide tips on how to approach certain poses or movements that can be challenging for beginners, so you feel more comfortable and knowledgeable before you start.

- If you smoke, exercise will present more of a challenge to your lungs and respiratory function. Once you become accustomed to a beginner's level and become moderately active, you may notice it takes more effort, which requires an increase in lung capacity and oxygen. Smoking will eventually present a challenge, and where quitting can be a long-term and difficult goal in itself, make an effort to cut back as much as it takes to allow your body's movements and exercise to continue. In time, you may find quitting becomes easier and more achievable than expected!

Once you get into a basic routine, there is a wide variety of individual and team activities to consider for your life. If you are a social person, joining a baseball team or badminton club may be ideal. For more solitary options, consider swimming, cycling, or jogging. Many gyms and community centers provide monthly plans and may offer a free trial period to see if their facilities work for you. This is a great opportunity to try new classes and equipment to gauge how much you can achieve, even if in the early stages of exercise, so that you can decide whether to pursue dance aerobics, spin classes, and/or weight training. Some gyms will provide a free consultation with a personal trainer to set a simple plan towards weight loss and strength training goals.

Food To Avoid

If you are on Renal diet, the items mentioned below should be avoided or used in moderation.

1. Soda in A Dark Color

Sodas contain additives that accommodate phosphorus in addition to sugar and calories, especially dark-colored sodas.

Phosphorus is often used in food and beverage processing to increase flavor, prolong shelf life, and avoid discoloration.

This extra phosphorus is absorbed more readily by the body than natural, animal and plant-based phosphorus.

Phosphorus in the form of chemicals isn't really bound to protein—with the exception of natural phosphorus—rather, it comes in the form of salt and is easily absorbed by the digestive tract.

In certain cases, additive phosphorus can be found in a product's ingredient list. Meat manufacturers, on the other hand, are not permitted to show the exact amount of phosphorus additives on the food label.

Although the amount of additive phosphorus varies depending on the type of beverage, most dark-colored sodas are expected to contain 50-100 mg per 200 ml serving. As a result, on a Renal diet sodas, particularly dark sodas, must be shunned.

2. Avocado

Avocados are known for their heart-healthy fiber, fats, and antioxidants, as well as their other nutritional benefits. Avocados are usually a healthy count to a diet, but people with kidney disease must elude them.

Avocados have a high potassium content, so they are a good source of potassium. They contain a monstrous 727 mg (per cup) of potassium (150 g). That is double the potassium a banana of medium size has. One cup of avocado provides nearly 37% of the 2,000 mg potassium restriction.

Avocados, like guacamole, must be eluded on Renal diet, particularly if you've been advised to limit your potassium intake.

3. Foods in Cans

Canned foods, such as soups, tomatoes, and beans, are often purchased due to their low cost and flexibility. On the other hand, many canned foods include a lot of sodium, which is added as a preservative to extend their shelf life.

Because of the sodium content in canned products, it is recommended that people with kidney disease prevent or limit their consumption. Low sodium or "no salt added" alternatives are normally better choices. Furthermore, draining and rinsing canned foods, such as canned beans and tuna, can lessen sodium content by 33 to 80 %, depending on the commodity.

To limit overall sodium consumption, it is normally safest to avoid, ban, or purchase low-sodium alternatives.

4. Bread Made from Whole Wheat

Choosing the best bread for those with kidney failure can be difficult.

Whole wheat bread is a more nutritious alternative, due to its higher fiber quality. However, white bread is usually recommended over whole-wheat for people with kidney disease. This is due to the phosphorus and potassium content. The more bran and whole grains in the bread, the higher the phosphorus and potassium content.

For e.g., a 1-ounce (30-gram) serving of whole wheat bread contains about 57 mg phosphorus and 69 mg potassium. In addition, white bread contains just 28 mg of potassium and phosphorus. It's worth noting that most bread and bread products, whether white or whole wheat, contain relatively high levels of sodium. It is in your best interests to read the nutrient labels of various types of bread, choose a lower sodium substitute if possible, and keep track of your serving sizes.

To reiterate, when you are on Renal diet, it is best practice to favor white bread, and compare the food labeling in order to choose a brand that contains lower sodium.

5. Rice (Brown)

Brown rice, like whole-wheat flour, is a whole grain with a higher potassium and phosphorus content than white rice. A cup of cooked brown rice contains 150 mg of phosphorus and 154 mg of potassium, while a cup of white rice contains just 69 mg of phosphorus and 54 mg of potassium (cooked).

White rice can be used in Renal diet to avoid an excessive intake of potassium and phosphorus, but only if the level is regulated and matched with other foods. Bulgur, pearled barley, buckwheat, and couscous are low-phosphorus grains that can be used as a substitute for brown rice.

6. Bananas

The potassium concentration of bananas is well recognized. Despite being inherently low in sodium, one medium banana provides 422 mg of potassium. If you eat a banana every day, sticking to a maximum potassium intake of 2,000 mg can be difficult.

Unfortunately, several other tropical fruits have high potassium levels as well. Pineapples, on the other hand, contain somewhat less potassium than most other tropical fruits and may be a more suitable yet delicious alternative.

On Renal diet, bananas are an unhealthy source of potassium and should be avoided.

7. Dairy Products

Dairy products are high in proteins and vitamins. They're a good source of phosphorus and potassium, as well as a good source of protein. For e.g., 1 cup (240 ml) of whole milk contains 222 mg of phosphorus and 349 mg of potassium (18).

However, eating too much dairy in comparison to other phosphorus-rich foods can be detrimental to bone health in those with kidney disease. This could come as a surprise given that dairy and milk are both recommended for strong bones and muscles.

However, consuming too much phosphorus causes an excess of phosphorus in the blood, weakening the kidneys and forcing calcium out of the bones. This will weaken and shorten bones over time, increasing the chance of fractures or breaks. Dairy foods are also high in protein, 1 cup (240 ml) of milk contains about 8 g of protein.

It may be important to limit dairy consumption in order to avoid the accumulation of protein wastes in the blood. Dairy replacements, such as unenriched rice milk and almond milk, are lower in calcium, protein and potassium than the milk of cows, making them a safer milk supplement while on a diet.

Dairy items have a lot of potassium, phosphate and protein, so they can be avoided if you are on Renal diet. Despite milk's calcium content (high), those with renal disease can experience bone loss due to its high phosphorus content.

8. Oranges and Orange Juice

While oranges and orange juice are probably best known for their vitamin C content, they are also high in potassium. One large orange has 333 mg of potassium (184 g). Furthermore, 1 cup of orange juice (240 ml) contains 473 mg of potassium. Oranges and orange juice can be avoided or restricted in the Renal diet due to their potassium content. Apples, strawberries and cranberries, as well as their juices, are ideal substitutes for oranges and orange juice due to their lower potassium content.

9. Meats That Have Been Processed

Processed meats have long been related to chronic diseases, and their high preservative content is commonly viewed as hazardous. Salted, cured, roasted, or frozen meats are examples of processed meats. Pepperoni, bacon, jerky and sausage are only a few examples.

Processed meat usually contains large amounts of salt, which is used to improve taste and conserve flavor. As a result, if processed meats are a big part of your diet, maintaining your daily sodium intake under 2,000 mg can be difficult. In addition, processed meat is a good source of protein. If you've been told to keep track of your protein consumption, you'll need to exclude refined meats from your diet.

Processed meats are high in protein and salt and should be consumed in moderation on Renal diet.

10. Pickles, Olives, And Relish

Significant amounts of salt are usually used during the pickling or curing period. A single pickle spear, for example, may contain over 300 mg of sodium. Similarly, 244 mg of sodium can be contained in 2 tablespoons of sweet pickle relish.

When processed olives are fermented and aged to make them less bitter, they also taste salty. 5 green pickled olives contain about 195 mg of sodium, which is a significant portion of the daily sodium intake in such a limited serving. Many supermarkets sell reduced-sodium pickles, olives, and relish, which have less sodium than regular versions.

Pickles, processed olives, and relish have a high salt level and should be avoided in the Renal diet.

11. Apricots

Apricots are high in vitamins C and A, as well as fiber. Though they are still a good source of potassium. The potassium content in a cup of fresh apricots is 427 mg. Potassium is also even more abundant in dried apricots. Over 1,500 mg potassium can be found in a cup of dried apricots (30).

That means that 75 % of the 2,000 mg potassium restriction can be met with only one cup of dried apricots. On Renal diet, apricots, particularly dried apricots, should be avoided.

They also have over 400 mg of caffeine per raw cup and over 1,500 mg of caffeine per dry cup, adding another reason as to why they should be avoided.

12. Sweet Potatoes and Potatoes

Potatoes and sweet potatoes, which are rich in potassium, can be leached or soaked to reduce their potassium content.

The potassium content of potatoes can also be reduced by half by cutting them into small, thin parts and boiling them for at least ten minutes. It has been found that potatoes that have been submerged in water for at least four hours lowered the amount of potassium. A potato has less potassium in it before boiling than those that have not been soaked. This method is known as the "double cook operation" or "potassium leaching."

While cooking potatoes twice decreases their potassium content, it's crucial to note that this method doesn't remove it entirely. Potassium levels can still be high in double-cooked potatoes, so portion control is advised to keep potassium levels under control.

13. Tomatoes

Tomatoes are another potassium-rich food that may not be appropriate for Renal diet. Tomatoes can be eaten raw or cooked, and sauces can be created with them, although a cup of tomato sauce has approximately 900 mg of potassium.

Tomatoes are widely used in some meals, which is unfortunate for those on Renal diet. Personal taste plays a big role in deciding on a potassium-free alternative. However, substituting tomato sauce for roasted red pepper sauce and consuming less potassium per meal can be just as delicious.

Tomatoes are another high-potassium snack to skip while you're on Renal diet.

14. Meals That Are Prepackaged, Ready-To-Eat, And Ready-To-Cook

Refined foods will add a significant amount of sodium to your diet. The most concentrated of all foods, packaged, premade and microwave meals, contain the highest sodium content.

Frozen pizza, instant noodles and microwaveable dinners are among the most important types to avoid. Maintaining a sodium level of up to 2,000 mg per day will be daunting if you consume heavily refined foods on a daily basis. Refined foods can be not only high in sodium, but they can also be poor in nutrients.

Packaged, instant, and premade meals are heavily processed diets with high sodium levels and nutritional deficiencies. These components should be kept to a minimum in a Renal diet.

15. Swiss Chard, Spinach, And Beet Greens

Leafy green vegetables including Swiss chard, spinach and beet greens are rich in a variety of nutrients and minerals, including potassium. Potassium content in a cup range from 140mg to 290 mg when served fresh. The potassium content of leafy vegetables reduces when cooked to a smaller serving size, but it remains stable when cooked to larger serving size.

When fried, half a cup of raw spinach, for example, can be reduced to around a tablespoon. As a result, half a cup of raw spinach has far more potassium than cooked spinach. To stop excess potassium, new Swiss chard, spinach and beet greens are preferred overcooked.

However, since these foods are high in oxalates, which can increase the risk of kidney stones in people who are prone to them, you should restrict their consumption. Kidney stones can exacerbate renal tissue injury and make it difficult for the kidneys to function properly.

16. Raisins, Dates and Prunes, To Name A Few.

Dried fruits such as dates, raisins and prunes are all common. All of the nutrients, including potassium, are concentrated as fruits are dried. For e.g., 1 cup of dried prunes contains 1,274 mg of potassium, nearly 5 times the potassium content of 1 cup of prunes when fresh.

In addition, only 4 dates contain 668 mg of potassium (42). If you're on a Renal diet, you should avoid these well-known dried fruits due to their high potassium level.

17. Pretzels, Popcorn and Crackers

Pretzels, popcorn and crackers are examples of ready-to-eat snack foods that are low in protein and high in salt. It's normal to consume more than the prescribed portion size of these ingredients, resulting in higher-than-expected salt intake. Furthermore, if potatoes are used to produce chips, they will have a high potassium content. It is best to avoid consuming these when on a Renal diet.

Kidney-Friendly Food

Many foods work well within the Renal diet. Once you see the available variety, it will not seem as restrictive or difficult to follow. The key is to focus on foods with a high level of nutrients, which make it easier for the kidneys to process the waste by not adding too much that the body needs to discard. Long-term renal function depends on maintaining and improving balance.

- **Garlic**: An excellent, vitamin-rich food for the immune system, garlic is a tasty substitute for salt in a variety of dishes. It acts as a significant source of vitamin C and B6, while aiding the kidneys in ridding the body of unwanted toxins. It's a great and healthy way to add flavor to skillet meals, pasta, soups, and stews.

- **Berries**: All berries are considered a good renal diet food due to their high level of fiber, antioxidants, and delicious taste, making them an easy option to include as a light snack or as an ingredient in smoothies, salads, and light desserts. Just one handful of blueberries can provide almost one day's vitamin C requirement, as well as a boost of fiber, which is good for weight loss and maintenance.

- **Bell peppers**: Flavorful and easy to enjoy both raw and cooked; bell peppers offer a good source of vitamin C, vitamin A, and fiber. Along with other kidney-friendly foods, they make the detoxification process much easier while boosting your body's nutrient level to prevent further health conditions and reduce existing deficiencies.

- **Onions**: This nutritious and tasty vegetable is excellent as a companion to garlic in many dishes or on its own. Like garlic, onions can provide flavor as an alternative to salt and provide a good source of vitamin C, vitamin B, manganese, and fiber, as well. Adding just one quarter or half of the onion is often enough for most meals because of its strong and pungent flavor.

- **Macadamia nuts**: If you enjoy nuts and seeds as snacks, you may learn that many contain high amounts of phosphorus and should be avoided or limited as much as possible. Fortunately, macadamia nuts are an easier option to digest and process, as they contain much lower amounts of phosphorus and make an excellent substitute for other nuts. They are a good source of other nutrients, as well, such as vitamin B, copper, manganese, iron, and healthy fats.

- **Pineapple**: Unlike other fruits that are high in potassium, a pineapple is an option that can be enjoyed more often than bananas and kiwis. Citrus fruits are generally high in potassium as well, so if you find yourself craving an orange or grapefruit, choose pineapple instead. In addition to providing high levels of vitamin B and fiber, pineapples can reduce inflammation thanks to an enzyme called bromelain.

- **Mushrooms**: In general, mushrooms are a safe and healthy option for the renal diet, especially the shiitake variety, high in nutrients such as selenium, vitamin B, and manganese. They contain a moderate amount of plant-based protein, which is easier for your body to digest and use than animal proteins. Shiitake and portobello mushrooms are often used in vegan diets as a meat substitute due to their texture and pleasant flavor.

Grocery List

Meat and Meat Substitutes

Beef
Chicken
Eggs
Egg substitute
Fish
Lamb
Pork, chops/ roast
Tofu
Tuna, canned
Turkey
Veal

Vegetables

Alfalfa sprouts
Arugula
Asparagus
Bean sprouts
Beets, canned
Cabbage, green/red
Carrots
Cauliflower
Celery
Chiles
Chives
Coleslaw
Corn
Cucumber
Eggplant
Endive
Ginger root
Green beans
Lettuce
Onions
Parsley
Radishes
Spaghetti squash
Turnips
Vegetables, mixed
Water chestnuts, canned

Fruits

Apple juice
Apples
Applesauce
Apricot nectar
Apricots, canned
Blackberries
Cherries
Cranberries
Cranberry juice
Cranberry sauce
Figs, fresh
Fruit cocktail
Grapefruit
Grapefruit juice
Grapes
Lemon
Lime
Peaches
Peach nectar
Pear nectar
Pears, canned
Pineapple
Plums
Raspberries
Strawberries
Tangerines
Watermelon

Breads and Cereals

Bagels, plain/blueberry
Bread, white/French/Italian
Cereals, Kellogg's Corn Flakes
Cereals, Cheerios
Cereals, Corn Chex
Couscous
Crackers, unsalted
Dinner rolls
English muffins
Grits
Hamburger/hot dog rolls
Pasta
Melba toast
Noodles
Oyster crackers
Pita bread
Pretzels, unsalted
Rice, brown/white
Spaghetti
Tortillas

Fats

Butter
Canola oil
Cream cheese
Margarine
Mayonnaise

Miracle Whip
Nondairy creamers
Olive oil

Sweets

Animal crackers
Angel food cake
Candy corn
Chewing gum
Cotton candy
Crispy rice treats
Graham crackers
Gumdrops
Gummy bears
Hard candy
Hot Tamales candy
Jell-O
Jelly beans
Jolly Rancher
Lemon cake

Life Savers
Marshmallows
Newtons (fig, strawberry, apple, blueberry)
Pie (apple, berry, cherry, lemon, peach)
Pound cake
Rice cakes
Vanilla wafers

Beverages

7UP
Coffee
Cream soda
Fruit punch
Ginger ale
Grape soda
Hi-C
Lemon-lime soda
Lemonade

Orange soda
Root beer
Tea

Dairy and Dairy Alternatives

Almond milk
Coffee-mate
Mocha Mix
Rice Dream
Rich's Coffee Rich

Other

Apple butter
Corn syrup
Honey
Jam
Jelly
Maple syrup
Sugar, brown or white
Sugar, powdered

PHOSPHORUS TAB

	LOWER PHOSPHORUS	HIGHER PHOSPHORUS	HIGEST PHOSPHORUS
	To 150 mg.	151 to 200 mg.	201 or more mg.
Meat & Poultry 3 ounces dry, cooked or as stated	Beef, ground, extra lean 137 Beef, ground, regular 144 Duck, domestic, with skin 133	Beef, chuck roast 163 Beef, eye round 177 Beef, sirloin steak 186 Chicken, white 185 Chicken, dark 154 Lamb, kabobs, domestic 190 Lamb, leg, roast, domestic 162 Lamb, leg roast, New Zealand 186 Pork, fresh, lion ribs 142 Turkey, white 188 Turkey, dark 157	Beef, bottom round 217 Beefalo 213 Pork, fresh, leg roast 224 Pork, fresh, spareribs 192 Pork, fresh, boneless loin chop 203 Veal, cubes, stewed 203 Veal, rib roast 211
	To 150 mg.	151 to 200 mg.	201 or more mg.
Fish 3 ounces dry, cooked or as stated	Clams, raw 144 Cod, Atlantic 117 Grouper 121 Oysters, Eastern, raw/canned 118 Oysters, Pacific, raw 138 Shrimp, moist heat 116	Catfish, breaded, fried 183 Crab, blue, moist heat 175 Crab, Dungeness, moist heat 149 Lobster, moist heat 157 Mussels, blue, raw 168 Shrimp, breaded, fried 185 Shrimp canned 198 Snapper 171 Tuna, light, canned in water 158	Calamari, fried 213 Clams, moist 287 Crab, Alaska, moist heat 238 Flounder 246 Haddock 205 Halibut 242 Oysters, Eastern, cooked 236 Mussels, blue, cooked 242 Salmon, canned, Pink/red 279 Salmon, fresh, cooked 234 Scallops, breaded, fried 203 Sole 246 Swordfish 287 Tuna, white, canned in oil 227 Tuna, light, in oil 265
	To 100 mg.	101 to 150 mg.	201 or more mg.
Dairy & Eggs Portions as stated	Butter, 1 tbsp. 3 Cheese, bure, 1 ounce 53 Cheese, feta, 1 ounce 96 Cottage cheese, nonfat, ½ cup 76 Cream cheese, 1 ounce 30 Cream, half&half, 1 tbsp. 14 Egg white, 1 medium 4 Egg yolk, 1 medium 86 Ice cream, 10% fat, vanilla ½ cup 67 Sherbet, ½ cup 38 Sour cream, ½ cup 98	Cheese, blue, 1 ounce 110 Cheese, cheddar, 1 ounce 145 Cheese, mozzarella, 1 ounce 105 Cheese, provolone, 1 ounce 141 Cheese, Swiss, 1 ounce 171 Cottage cheese 4% fat, ½ cup 139 Cottage cheese 2% fat, ½ cup 170 Ice cream, soft serve, vanilla ½ cup 106	Buttermilk, 1 cup 219 Cheese, parmesan, 1 ounce 229 Cheese, ricotta, par skim, ½ cup 226 Milk, evaporated skim, ½ cup 248 Milk, no fat, 1 cup 247-275 Milk, Whole, 1 cup 228 Milk 1% low fat, 1 cup 235-273 Processed American Cheese, 1 ounce 211 Yogurt, skim, 1 cup 255 Yogurt, low fat, 1 cup 326 Yogurt, shole milk, 1 cup 215

	To 100 mg.	101 to 150 mg.	151 or more mg.
Legumes ½ cup cooked or as stated	Peas, split 97 Peanuts, boiled 63 Soy milk 59	Beans, black 120 Beans, black turtle 140 Beans, fava 106 Beans, kidney 125 Beans, lima, thick 104 Beans, lima, thin 116 Beans, navy 143 Beans, pinto 136 Black-eyed peas 134 Chickpeas 137 Peanut butter, 2 tbsps. 102 Tofu, raw, regular 120	Beans, small, white 152 Lentils 178 Peanuts, dry roasted, 2 ounces 200 Peanuts, oil roasted, 2 ounces 290 Soyabeans 211 Tofu, raw, firm 239
	To 65 mg.	66 to 150 mg.	151 or more mg.
Grains & Cereals Portions as stated	Bagel, plain, 3 ½" diameter, 1 46 Barley, pearled, cooked, ½ cup 43 Bread, pita, 6 ½" diameter, 1 60 Corn flakes, 1 cup 14 Couscous, cooked ½ cup 20 Crispy rice cereal, 1 cup 31 Farina, cooked, ¾ cup 21 Hominy grits, ½ cup 15 Rice, white, cooked, ½ cup 37	Bread, pumpernickel, 1 slice 71 Bread, shole wheat, 1 slice 66 English muffin, plain, one 67 Oatmeal, cooked, 1 packet 133 Pasta "al dente", 1 cup 85 Raisin bran, ½ cup 124 Rice, brown, cooked ½ cup 81 Shredded wheat, 1 large biscuit 86 Wheat flakes, 1 cup 100 Wheat flour, white 1 cup 135	Bran cereal, 100%, ½ cup 402 Corn flour, whole grain, 1 cup 318 Cornmeal, whole grain, 1 cup 294 Wheat flour, shole grain, 1 cup 415 Cheat germ, plain, 9 ¼ cup 324
	To 65 mg.	66 to 150 mg.	151 or more mg.
Snack & Sweets Portions as stated	Chestnuts, Chinese, canned, 2 ounces 10 Cookies, shortbread, 4 small 39 Gelatin, water base, ½ cup 23 Popcorn, air popped, 1 cup 22 Rice caked, one 34 Cool Whip, 2 tbsp. 0	Angel food cake, 1/12 91 Cocoa, dry, unsweetened, 2 tbsps. 74 Macadamia nuts, oil roast, 2 ounces 114	Almonds, oil/dry, 2 ounces 312 Cashews, dry roast, 2 ounces 278 Cashews, oil roast, 2 ounces, 242 Pecans, oil/dry roast, 2 ounces 170 Walnuts, black, 2 ounces 264 Walnuts, English, 2 ounces, 180

POTASSIUM TAB

	Higher Potassium Food	Lower Potassium Alternatives
Seasoning, Spreads/Butter, Sauces	- Peanut butter - Chocolate spread - Brown sauce - Tomato ketchup - Tomato puree, pasta - Marmite/Bovril/Vegemite - Salt substitutes, Low Salt, So-Lo, low-sodium salt	- All herbs and spices - Pepper - All chili sauces, curry powder - Garlic - Vinegar - Mayonnaise lite
Savoury Snacks	- Potato/root vegetable crisps - Nuts - Seeds	- Corn/maize snacks (e.g tortilla chips) - Rice snacks - Wheat snacks - Popcorn, pretzels, bread sticks - Cream crackers, crispbreads
Sweet Foods	If you have diabetes, you may need to limit your intake of sugar. Chocolate, Cocoa, Dried fruit, Coconut or nuts should be avoided	- Fruit pie/Crumble - Jelly - Plain biscuits (digestive, Rich Tea, Maire..) - Boiled/chewy/jelly sweets, fruit pastilles - Marshmallows, homemade caramelized popcorn
Meat, Fish and Vegetarian Alternatives	- Nuts - Seeds - Organ and red meat	- Poultry - Fish and seafood - Eggs
Carbohydrates	- Steamed, jacket or instant mashed potatoes - Frozen, oven, microwave, chip shop chips - Manufactured potato products (e.g. hash browns, potato waffles, potato croquettes..) - Breads containing nuts, seed, dried fruits - Naan bread (limit to 80g per day) - Cereals containing bran, dried fruit, nuts and chocolate e.g. muesli - All Bran, Bran Buds, Sultana Bran, Weetos, Fruit and Fibre, Grape Nuts, Chocolate Crisp	- White bread – 2.8/3.5 oz. per day (2 slices) - Whole meal bread of rolls - 1.5 slices - Pita bread – 2 nos - Rice – 2 cups - Pasta/Noodles – 1.5 oz. dry weight - Couscous – 3.5 oz. - Sago – 3.5 oz. - Millets

Vegetables	<ul><li>Asparagus</li><li>Artichoke</li><li>Aubergine</li><li>Baked Beans</li><li>Beetroot</li><li>Broad beans</li><li>Brussels sprouts</li><li>Celery</li><li>Okra</li><li>Parsnips</li><li>Spinach</li><li>Dried Vegetables</li><li>Mushrooms</li><li>Sweetcorn</li><li>Tomatoes</li></ul>	<ul><li>Beansprouts – 4 tbsps.</li><li>Broccoli – 2 spears</li><li>Cabbage – 2 handfuls</li><li>Carrots – 3 tbsps.</li><li>Cauliflower – 6 florets</li><li>Cucumber – 3.5 oz.</li><li>French beans – 3 tbsps.</li><li>Lettuce – 1 small bowl</li><li>Marrow – 3 tbsps.</li><li>Peas, boiled – 3 tbsps.</li><li>Peppers ½</li><li>Runners beans – 3 tbsps.</li></ul>
Fruits	<ul><li>Apricots</li><li>Avocado</li><li>Bananas</li><li>Blackcurrants</li><li>Mango</li><li>Orange</li><li>Cantaloupe/honeydew melon</li><li>Coconut</li><li>Figs</li><li>Gooseberries</li><li>Prunes</li><li>Rhubarb</li><li>Lychees</li><li>Star fruit</li><li>All dry fruit (e.g; raisin, sultanas, prunes, dates)</li><li>All fruits juices</li></ul>	<ul><li>Apple – 1 cup</li><li>Peach – 2.4 oz.</li><li>Pear – 3.5 oz.</li><li>Pineapple – 1 slice</li><li>Clementine/mandarin/satsuma/tangerine – 3.5 oz.</li><li>Plum – 3.5 oz.</li><li>Blueberries – 3.5 oz.</li><li>Cherries – 2.8 oz.</li><li>Strawberries – 3.5 oz.</li><li>Raspberries – 80g</li><li>Grapefruit – 3.5 oz.</li></ul>

Breakfast

1. Fast Microwave Egg Scramble

Preparation time: 5 minutes
Cooking time: 1-2 minutes
Servings: 2

INGREDIENTS:

- 1 large egg
- 2 large egg whites
- 2 tablespoons of milk
- Kosher pepper, ground

DIRECTIONS:

1. Spray a coffee cup with a bit of cooking spray.
2. Whisk all the ingredients together and place into the coffee cup.
3. Place the cup with the eggs into the microwave and set to cook for approx. 45 seconds. Take out and stir.
4. Cook it for another 30 seconds after returning it to the microwave.
5. Serve.

Nutrition: Calories: 128.6 kcal Carbohydrate: 2.47 g Protein: 12.96 g Sodium: 286.36 mg Potassium: 185.28 mg Phosphorus: 122.22 mg Dietary fiber: 0 g Fat: 5.96 g

2. Raspberry Overnight Porridge

Preparation Time: 5 minutes
Cooking Time: Overnight
Servings: 2

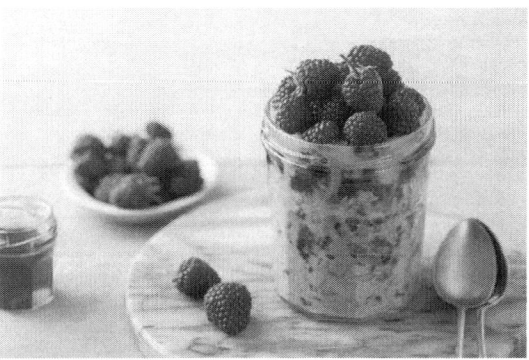

INGREDIENTS:

- 1/3 cup of rolled oats
- 1/2 cup almond milk
- 1 tablespoon of honey
- 5 – 6 raspberries, fresh or canned and unsweetened

DIRECTIONS:

1. Combine the oats, almond milk, and honey in a mason jar and place it into the fridge overnight.
2. Serve the following morning with the raspberries on top.

Nutrition: Calories: 143.6 Carbohydrate: 34.62 g Protein: 3.44 g Sodium: 77.88 mg Potassium: 153.25 mg Phosphorus: 99.3 mg Dietary Fiber: 7.56 g Fat: 3.91 g

3. Summer Veggie Omelet

Preparation time: 5 minutes
Cooking time: 5 minutes
Servings: 2

INGREDIENTS:

- 4 large egg whites
- ¼ cup of sweet corn, frozen
- 1/3 cup of zucchini, grated

- 2 green onions, sliced
- 1 tablespoon of cream cheese
- Kosher pepper

DIRECTIONS:

1. Grease a medium pan with some cooking spray and add the onions, corn and grated zucchini.
2. Sauté for a couple of minutes until softened.
3. Beat the eggs together with the water, cream cheese, and pepper in a bowl.
4. Add the eggs into the veggie mixture in the pan and let cook while moving the edges from inside to outside with a spatula, to allow raw egg to cook through the edges.
5. Turn the omelet with the aid of a dish (placed over the pan and flipped upside down and then back to the pan).
6. Let sit for another 1-2 minutes.
7. Fold in half and serve.

Nutrition: Calories: 90 kcal Carbohydrate: 15.97 g Protein: 8.07 g Sodium: 227 mg Potassium: 244.24 mg Phosphorus: 45.32 mg Dietary fiber: 0.88 g Fat: 2.4 g

4. Yogurt Parfait with Strawberries

Preparation Time: 3 minutes
Cooking Time: 1 minute
Servings: 2

INGREDIENTS:

- 1/2 cup of soy yogurt (plain)
- 1 scoop of vanilla flavored protein
- 5 fresh strawberries, sliced
- 1 tablespoon of agave syrup

DIRECTIONS:

1. In a bowl, slowly whisk the protein powder with the yogurt.
2. Add the strawberry slices and the agave syrup on top.
3. Serve.

Nutrition: Calories: 153.25 Carbohydrate: 23.5 g Protein: 12.67 g Sodium: 93.32 mg Potassium: 85.9 mg Phosphorus: 62.75 mg Dietary Fiber: 1.43 g Fat: 1.17 g

5. Apple and Onion Omelet

Preparation Time: 10 minutes
Cooking Time: 20 minutes
Servings: 2

INGREDIENTS:

- ¾ cup sweet onion, sliced
- 1 large apple peeled, cored, sliced
- 1 tablespoon unsalted butter
- 3 eggs
- 1/8 teaspoon ground black pepper
- 1 tablespoon water
- ¼ cup milk, low-fat
- 2 tablespoons shredded cheddar cheese, low-fat

DIRECTIONS:

1. Switch on the oven, then set it to 400ºF and let it preheat. Crack eggs in a bowl, add black pepper and water, and whisk until beaten.
2. Take a small heatproof skillet pan, place it over medium heat, add butter and when it melts, add onions and apple and cook for 6 minutes until sauted. Spread onion-

apple mixture evenly, pour egg mixture over it, spread evenly, and cook for 2 minutes until eggs begin to set. Then sprinkle cheese on top of eggs, transfer skillet pan into the heated oven, and bake for 12 minutes or until omelet has set. When done, remove the pan from the oven, cut the omelet in half, distribute it between two plates, and then serve.

Nutrition: Calories 282 Fat 16 g Protein 13 g Carbohydrates 22 g Fiber 3.5 g

6. Apple Cherry Breakfast Risotto

Preparation Time: 10 minutes
Cooking Time: 15 minutes
Servings: 2

INGREDIENTS:

- 2 large apples, cored and chopped
- 1 ½ cups Arborio rice
- ½ cup dried cherries
- 1 ½ teaspoon cinnamon
- 2 tablespoons butter
- ¼ teaspoon salt
- 1 cup apple juice
- 3 cups of milk

DIRECTIONS:

1. Add butter to the pressure-cooking pot and heat for 2 to 3 minutes.
2. Whisk in the rice, continue heating, and consistently whisk until rice darkens for about 3 to 4 minutes.
3. Put the spices, brown sugar, and apples.
4. Whisk in the juice and milk.
5. Set pressure cooker to high pressure and select 6 minutes cook time and heat.
6. Once the timer beeps, unplug the cooker and use a fast pressure release to release the pressure.
7. Gently remove the lid of the pressure cooker and whisk in dried cherries.
8. Serve hot, and garnish with extra sliced almonds, brown sugar, and milk.

Nutrition: Calories: 258 Fat: 3g Carbs: 50g Protein: 10g Sodium: 227mg Potassium: 580mg Phosphorus: 150mg

7. Breakfast Burrito

Preparation Time: 10 minutes
Cooking Time: 3 minutes
Servings: 2 burritos

INGREDIENTS:

- 3 tablespoons green chiles, diced
- ½ teaspoon hot pepper sauce
- ¼ teaspoon ground cumin
- 4 eggs
- 2 flour tortillas, burrito size

DIRECTIONS:

1. Take a medium-sized skillet pan, place it over medium heat, grease it with oil, and let it get hot.
2. Crack eggs in a bowl, add chilies, hot sauce, and cumin, whisk until combined, then pour the egg mixture in the hot skillet and cook for 2 minutes, or until eggs have been cooked to the desired level.

3. Meanwhile, heat the tortillas by microwaving them for 20 seconds until hot.
4. When eggs have cooked, distribute evenly between hot tortillas and roll it up like a burrito.
5. Serve straight away.

Nutrition: Calories 366 Fat 18 g Protein 18 g Carbohydrates 33 g Fiber 2.5 g

8. Mushroom and Red Pepper Omelet

Preparation Time: 5 minutes
Cooking Time: 12 minutes
Servings: 2 plates

INGREDIENTS:
- 2 tablespoons white onion, diced
- ¼ cup sweet red peppers, diced
- ½ cup mushrooms, diced
- ¼ teaspoon ground black pepper
- 1 teaspoon Worcestershire sauce
- 2 teaspoons unsalted butter
- 3 eggs
- 2 tablespoons whipped cream cheese

DIRECTIONS:

1. Take a medium-sized skillet pan, place it over medium heat, add 1 teaspoon butter and when it melts, add onions and mushrooms and cook for 5 minutes, or until onions are tender.
2. Stir in red pepper, then transfer vegetables to a plate and set aside until needed.
3. Crack the eggs in a bowl, add Worcestershire sauce, and whisk until combined.
4. Return skillet pan over medium heat, add remaining butter and when it melts, pour in the egg mixture, and cook for 2 minutes, or until omelet is partially cooked.
5. Then top cooked vegetables on one side of the omelet, top with cream cheese, and continue cooking until omelet is cooked completely.
6. When done, remove the pan from the heat, cover the filling of the omelet by folding the other half of the omelet, sprinkle it with black pepper, and then divide omelet into two.
7. Serve straight away.

Nutrition: Calories 199 Fat 15 g Protein 11 g Carbohydrates 4 g Fiber 0.6 g

9. Mexican Scrambled Eggs in Tortilla

Preparation Time: 5 minutes
Cooking Time: 2 minutes
Servings: 2

INGREDIENTS:
- 2 medium corn tortillas
- 4 egg whites
- 1 teaspoons cumin
- 3 teaspoons green chilies, diced
- ½ teaspoons hot pepper sauce
- 2 tablespoons salsa
- ½ teaspoons salt

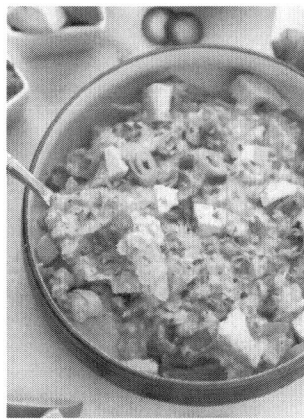

DIRECTIONS:

1. Spray some cooking spray on a medium skillet and heat for a few seconds.
2. Whisk the eggs with the green chilies, hot sauce, and comminute
3. Add the eggs into the pan, and whisk with a spatula to scramble. Add the salt.
4. Cook until fluffy and done (1-2 minutes) over low heat.
5. Open the tortillas and spread 1 tablespoon salsa on each.
6. Distribute the egg mixture onto the tortillas and wrap gently to make a burrito.
7. Serve warm.

Nutrition: Calories: 44.1 kcal Carbohydrate: 2.23 g Protein: 7.69 g Sodium: 854 mg Potassium: 189 mg

10. Mexican Style Burritos

Preparation Time: 5 minutes
Cooking Time: 15 minutes
Servings: 2
INGREDIENTS:

- Olive oil – 1 tablespoon
- Corn tortillas – 2
- Red onion – ¼ cup, chopped
- Red bell peppers – ¼ cup, chopped
- Red chili – ½, deseeded and chopped
- Eggs – 2
- Juice of 1 lime
- Cilantro – 1 tablespoon chopped

DIRECTIONS:

1. Turn the broiler to medium heat and place the tortillas underneath for 1 to 2 minutes on each side or until lightly toasted.
2. Remove and keep the broiler on.
3. Sauté onion, chili and bell peppers for 5 to 6 minutes or until soft.
4. Place the eggs on top of the onions and peppers and place skillet under the broiler for 5-6 minutes or until the eggs are cooked.
5. Serve half the eggs and vegetables on top of each tortilla and sprinkle with cilantro and lime juice to serve.

Nutrition: Calories: 202 Fat: 13g Carbohydrate: 19g Phosphorus: 184mg Potassium: 233mg Sodium: 77mg Protein: 9g

11. Buckwheat and Grapefruit Porridge

Preparation Time: 5 minutes
Cooking Time: 20 minutes
Servings: 2
INGREDIENTS:

- Buckwheat – ½ cup
- Grapefruit – ¼, chopped
- Honey – 1 tablespoon
- Almond milk – 1 ½ cups

- Water – 2 cups

DIRECTIONS:

1. Boil water on the stove. Add the buckwheat and place the lid on the pan.
2. Simmer for 7 to 10 minutes, in a low heat. Check to ensure water does not dry out.
3. Remove and set aside for 5 minutes, do this when most of the water is absorbed.
4. Drain excess water from the pan and stir in almond milk, heating through for 5 minutes.
5. Add the honey and grapefruit.
6. Serve.

Nutrition: Calories: 231 Fat: 4g Carbohydrate: 43g Phosphorus: 165mg Potassium: 370mg Sodium: 135mg

12. Vegetable Omelet

Preparation time: 15 minutes
Cooking time: 10 minutes
Servings: 3

INGREDIENTS:

- Egg whites – 4
- Egg – 1
- Chopped fresh parsley – 2 Tbsps.
- Water – 2 Tbsps.
- Olive oil spray
- Chopped and boiled red bell pepper – ½ cup
- Chopped scallion – ¼ cup, both green and white parts
- Ground black pepper

DIRECTIONS:

1. Whisk together the egg, egg whites, parsley, and water until well blended. Set aside.
2. Spray a skillet with olive oil spray and place over medium heat.
3. Sauté the peppers and scallion for 3 minutes or until softened.
4. Pour the egg mixture into the skillet over vegetables and cook, swirling the skillet, for 2 minutes or until the edges start to set. Cook until set.
5. Season with black pepper and serve.

Nutrition: Calories: 77 Fat: 3g Carbohydrate: 2g Phosphorus: 67mg Potassium: 194mg Sodium: 229mg Protein: 12g

13. Feta Mint Omelet

Preparation time: 10 minutes
Cooking time: 5 minutes
Servings: 1

INGREDIENTS:

- 3 eggs
- 1/4 cup fresh mint, chopped
- 2 tablespoon coconut milk
- 1/2 tablespoon olive oil
- 2 tablespoon feta cheese, crumbled
- Pepper to taste
- Salt to taste

DIRECTIONS:

1. In a bowl, whisk eggs with feta cheese, mint, milk, pepper, and salt.
2. Heat olive oil in a pan over low heat. Pour egg mixture into the pan and cook until eggs are set.

3. Flip omelet and cook for 2 minutes more.
4. Serve and enjoy.

<u>Nutrition</u>: Calories: 275cal Fat: 20g Carbohydrate: 4g Sugar: 4g Protein: 20g Cholesterol: 505mg

14. Pumpkin Apple Muffins

Preparation time: 10 minutes
Cooking time: 20 minutes
Serving: 2

INGREDIENTS:

- 1/2 cup diced cored and peeled apple
- 1 teaspoon vanilla
- 1 egg
- 1/4 cup olive oil
- 1/4 cup honey
- 1 cup pumpkin puree
- 2 teaspoon Phosphorus-Free baking powder
- 1 cup wheat bran
- 1 cup plain flour

DIRECTIONS:

1. Warm the oven to 350°F. Take a cupcake tin and place a paper liner into each cup.
2. Add baking powder, wheat bran, and flour into a medium bowl. Stir to mix well.
3. Add the vanilla, egg, olive oil, honey, and pumpkin to a small bowl and combine.
4. Mix the pumpkin mixture into the dry ingredients.
5. Add in the apple and stir to combine.
6. Spoon batter into muffin papers. Don't overfill.
7. Bake for 20 minutes. Once over, stick a toothpick in the middle. If it comes out clean, it means they are done. Serve and enjoy!

<u>Nutrition</u>: Calories: 125 Protein: 2 g Sodium: 8 mg Potassium: 177 mg Phosphorus: 120 mg

15. Feta And Bell Pepper Quiche

Preparation time: 10 minutes
Cooking time: 20 minutes
Serving: 2

INGREDIENTS:

- Pepper, to taste
- 2 tablespoons chopped basil
- 1/4 cup low sodium feta cheese
- 1/4 cup plain flour
- 4 eggs
- 1 cup unsweetened rice milk
- 1 chopped bell pepper
- 1 teaspoon minced garlic
- 1 small chopped sweet onion
- 1 teaspoon olive oil plus more

DIRECTIONS:

1. Warm your oven to 400°F. Brush a small amount of olive oil into a 9-inch pie pan.
2. Warm the oil in a skillet on medium heat.
3. Cook the onion and garlic until they become soft.
1. Add in bell pepper and cook for another 3 minutes.
4. Place the vegetables into the pie plate that has been brushed with olive oil.
5. Place the eggs, flour, and rice milk in a medium bowl and combine until smooth.

6. Add in the basil and feta, then sprinkle with pepper. Stir well to combine.
7. Pour eggs over the vegetables in the pie plate.
8. Bake until the edges are golden brown, and the center is just set. This should take about 20 minutes.
9. This can be served cold, room temperature, or hot. Enjoy!

Nutrition: Calories: 172 Protein: 8 g Sodium: 154 mg Potassium: 122 mg Phosphorus: 120 mg

16. Quinoa Porridge

Preparation time: 10 minutes
Cooking time: 0 minutes
Serving: 2

INGREDIENTS:

- 1 cup cashew milk, warm
- 1 cup blueberries
- 2 cups quinoa, cooked
- ¼ cup chopped walnuts, toasted
- 2 teaspoons raw honey
- ½ teaspoon ground cinnamon
- 1 tablespoon chia seeds

DIRECTIONS:

1. In a bowl, mix the cashew milk with the blueberries, quinoa, walnuts, honey, cinnamon, and chia seeds. Stir well, divide into 2 small bowls and serve. Enjoy!

Nutrition: Calories: 151 Fat: 2 g Fiber: 11 g Carbohydrate: 14 g Protein: 13 g

17. Egg and Veggie Muffins

Preparation Time: 15 minutes
Cooking Time: 20 minutes
Servings: 4

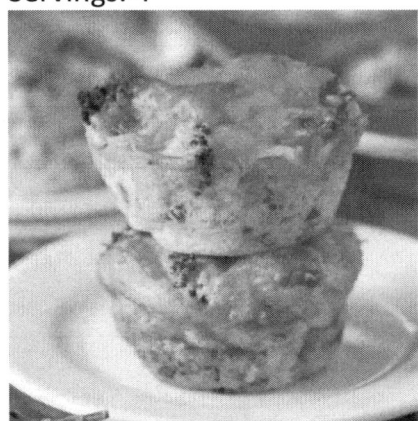

INGREDIENTS:

- 4 Eggs
- 2 tablespoons unsweetened rice milk
- ½ chopped sweet onion
- ½ chopped red bell pepper
- Pinch red pepper flakes
- Pinch ground black pepper

DIRECTIONS:

1. Preheat the oven to 350°F.
2. Spray 4 muffin pans with cooking spray. Set aside.
3. Whisk the milk, eggs, onion, red pepper, parsley, red pepper flakes, and black pepper until mixed.
4. Pour the egg mixture into prepared muffin pans.
5. Bake until the muffins are puffed and golden, about 18 to 20 minutes. Serve.

Nutrition: Calories: 84 Fat: 5g Carbohydrate: 3g Protein: 7g Sodium: 75mg Potassium: 117mg Phosphorus: 110mg

18. Berry Chia with Yogurt

Preparation Time: 35 minutes

Cooking Time: 5 minutes

Servings: 2

INGREDIENTS:

- ½ cup chia seeds, dried
- 2 cup Plain yogurt
- 1/3 cup strawberries, chopped
- ¼ cup blackberries
- ¼ cup raspberries
- 4 teaspoons Splenda

DIRECTIONS:

1. Mix up together Plain yogurt with Splenda and chia seeds.
2. Transfer the mixture into the serving ramekins (jars) and leave for 35 minutes.
3. After this, add blackberries, raspberries, and strawberries. Mix up the meal well.
4. Serve it immediately or store it in the fridge for up to 2 days.

Nutrition: Calories: 150 Fat: 5g Carbohydrate: 19g Protein: 6.8g Sodium: 65mg Potassium: 226mg Phosphorus: 75mg

19. Arugula Eggs with Chili Peppers

Preparation Time: 7 minutes

Cooking Time: 10 minutes

Servings: 2

INGREDIENTS:

- 2 cups arugula, chopped
- 3 eggs, beaten
- ½ chili pepper, chopped
- 1 tablespoon butter
- 1 oz Parmesan, grated

DIRECTIONS:

1. Toss butter in the skillet and melt it.
2. Add arugula and sauté it over medium heat for 5 minutes. Stir it from time to time.
3. Meanwhile, mix up together Parmesan, chili pepper, and eggs.
4. Pour the egg mixture over the arugula and scramble well.
5. Cook for 5 minutes more over medium heat.

Nutrition: Calories: 218 Fat: 15g Carbohydrate: 2.8g Protein: 17g Sodium: 656mg Potassium: 243mg Phosphorus: 310mg

20. Eggplant Chicken Sandwich

Preparation Time: 10 minutes

Cooking Time: 15 minutes

Servings: 2

INGREDIENTS:

- 1 eggplant, trimmed
- 10 oz chicken fillet
- 1 teaspoon Plain yogurt
- ½ teaspoon minced garlic
- 1 tablespoon fresh cilantro, chopped
- 2 lettuce leaves
- 1 teaspoon olive oil
- ½ teaspoon salt
- ½ teaspoon chili pepper
- 1 teaspoon butter

DIRECTIONS:

1. Slice the eggplant lengthwise into 4 slices.
2. Rub the eggplant slices with minced garlic and brush with olive oil.
3. Grill the eggplant slices on the preheated to 375F grill for 3 minutes from each side.
4. Meanwhile, rub the chicken fillet with salt and chili pepper.
5. Place it in the skillet and add butter.
6. Roast the chicken for 6 minutes from each side over medium-high heat.
7. Cool the cooked eggplants gently and spread one side of them with Plain yogurt.
8. Add lettuce leaves and chopped fresh cilantro.
9. After this, slice the cooked chicken fillet and add over the lettuce.
10. Cover it with the remaining sliced eggplant to get the sandwich shape. Pin the sandwich with the toothpick if needed.

Nutrition: Calories: 276 Fat: 11g Carbohydrate: 41g Protein: 13.8g Sodium: 775mg Potassium: 532mg Phosphorus: 187mg

21. Grandma's Pancake Special

Preparation Time: 5 minutes
Cooking Time: 15 minutes
Servings: 2

INGREDIENTS:

- 1 tablespoon oil
- 1 cup milk
- 1 egg
- 2 teaspoons sodium free baking powder
- 2 tablespoons sugar
- 1 ¼ cups flour

DIRECTIONS :

1. Mix together all the dry ingredients such as the flour, sugar and baking powder.
2. Combine oil, milk and egg in another bowl. Once done, add them all to the flour mixture.
3. Make sure that as your stir the mixture, blend them together until slightly lumpy.
4. In a hot greased griddle, pour-in at least ¼ cup of the batter to make each pancake.
5. To cook, ensure that the bottom is a bit brown, then turn and cook the other side, as well.

Nutrition: Calories: 167 Carbohydrate: 50g Protein: 11g Fats: 11g Phosphorus: 176mg Potassium: 215mg Sodium: 70mg

Salads

22. Thai Cucumber Salad

Preparation Time: 5 minutes
Cooking Time: 5 minutes
Servings: 2

INGREDIENTS:

- ¼ cup chopped Macadamia Nuts
- ¼ cup white sugar
- ½ cup cilantro
- ¼ cup rice wine vinegar
- 3 cucumbers
- 2 jalapeno peppers

DIRECTIONS:

1. In a bowl add all ingredients and mix well
2. Serve with dressing

Nutrition: Calories: 20 Fat: 0g Sodium: 85mg Carbohydrate: 5g Protein: 1g Potassium: 190.4 mg Phosphorus: 46.8mg

23. Butterscotch Apple Salad

Preparation Time: 8 minutes
Cooking Time: 1 hour
Servings: 6

INGREDIENTS:

- 3 cups jazz apples, chopped
- 8 oz. canned crushed pineapple
- 8 oz. whipped topping
- 1/2 cup butterscotch topping
- 1/3 cup almonds
- 1/4 cup butterscotch chips

DIRECTIONS:

1. Put all the salad ingredients into a suitable salad bowl.
2. Mix well and refrigerate for 1 hour.
3. Serve.

Nutrition: Calories: 293 Fat: 12.7g Sodium: 152mg Phosphorous: 202mg Potassium: 296mg Carbohydrate: 45.5g Dietary Fiber: 4.2g Protein: 4.2g

24. Grapes Jicama Salad

Preparation Time: 5 minutes
Cooking time: 0 minutes
Servings: 2

INGREDIENTS:

- 1 jicama, peeled and sliced
- 1 carrot, sliced
- 1/2 medium red onion, sliced
- 1 ¼ cup seedless grapes
- 1/3 cup fresh basil leaves
- 1 tablespoon apple cider vinegar
- 1 ½ tablespoon lemon juice
- 1 ½ tablespoon lime juice

DIRECTIONS:

1. Put all the salad ingredients into a suitable salad bowl.
2. Toss them well and refrigerate for 1 hour.
3. Serve.

Nutrition: Calories: 203 Total Fat: 0.7g Saturated Fat: 0.2g Cholesterol: 0mg Sodium: 44mg Carbohydrate: 48.2g Dietary Fiber: 18.4g Sugars: 19.1g Protein: 3.7g Calcium: 79mg Phosphorous: 141mg Potassium: 429mg

25. Pineapple Berry Salad

Preparation Time: 10 minutes
Cooking Time: 5 minutes
Servings: 4

INGREDIENTS:

- 4 cups pineapple, peeled and cubed
- 3 cups strawberries, chopped
- 1/4 cup honey
- 1/2 cup basil leaves
- 1 tablespoon lemon zest
- 1/2 cup blueberries

DIRECTIONS:

1. Prepare a salad bowl.
2. Put all the ingredients.
3. Mix well and serve.

Nutrition: Calories: 128 Fat: 0.6g Sodium: 3mg Phosphorous: 151mg Potassium: 362mg Carbohydrate: 33.1g Protein: 1.8g

26. Carrot Jicama Salad

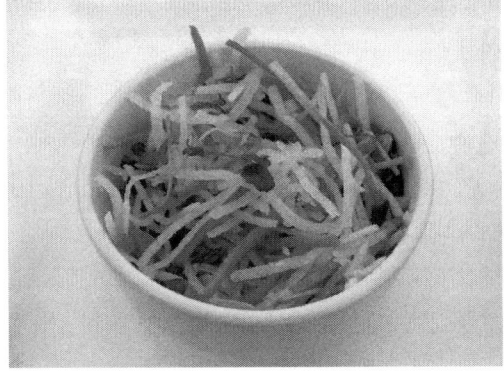

Preparation Time: 5 minutes
Cooking time: 0 minutes
Servings: 2

INGREDIENTS:

- 2 cup carrots, julienned
- 1 1/2 cups jicama, julienned
- 2 tablespoons lime juice
- 1 tablespoon olive oil
- ½ tablespoon apple cider
- ½ teaspoon brown Swerve

DIRECTIONS:

1. Put all the salad ingredients into a suitable salad bowl.
2. Toss them well and refrigerate for 1 hour.
3. Serve.

Nutrition: Calories: 173 Total Fat: 7.1g Saturated Fat: 0.5g Cholesterol: 0mg Sodium: 80mg Carbohydrate: 20.7g Dietary Fiber: 5.9g Sugars: 7.7g Protein: 1.6g Calcium: 50mg Phosphorous: 96mg Potassium: 501mg

27. Balsamic Beet Salad

Preparation Time: 5 minutes
Cooking time: 0 minutes
Servings: 2

INGREDIENTS:

- 1 cucumber, peeled and sliced
- 15 oz. canned low-sodium beets, sliced
- 4 teaspoon balsamic vinegar
- 2 teaspoon sesame oil
- 2 tablespoons Gorgonzola cheese

DIRECTIONS:

1. Take a suitable salad bowl.
2. Start tossing in all the ingredients.
3. Mix well and serve.

Nutrition: Calories: 145 Total Fat: 7.8g Saturated Fat: 2.4g Cholesterol: 10mg Sodium: 426mg Carbohydrate: 16.4g Dietary Fiber: 3.8g Sugars: 11.1g Protein: 5g Calcium: 109mg Phosphorous: 79mg Potassium: 229mg

28. Carrot Zucchini Salad

Preparation Time: 5 minutes

Cooking time: 0 minutes

Servings: 2

INGREDIENTS:

- 1/4 cup unseasoned rice vinegar
- 1/8 teaspoon stevia
- 1/2 teaspoon olive oil
- 1/8 teaspoon black pepper
- 1/2 zucchini, peeled and julienned
- 1 cup carrots, julienned
- 2 tablespoons red bell pepper, julienned

DIRECTIONS:

1. Take a suitable salad bowl.
2. Start tossing in all the ingredients.
3. Mix well and serve.

Nutrition: Calories: 92 Total Fat: 1.6g Saturated Fat: 0.2g Cholesterol: 0mg Sodium: 43mg Carbohydrate: 6.1g Dietary Fiber: 3.5g Sugars: 3.7g Protein: 2.3g Calcium: 45mg Phosphorous: 147mg Potassium: 529mg

29. Broccoli Lettuce Salad

Preparation Time: 5 minutes

Cooking time: 0 minutes

Servings: 2

INGREDIENTS:

- 1 cup lettuce, chopped
- ¼ zucchini, peeled and cubed
- 4 carrots, diced
- 1/4 cup broccoli florets
- 2 tablespoons balsamic vinegar
- 1 teaspoon olive oil

DIRECTIONS:

1. Take a suitable salad bowl.
2. Start tossing in all the ingredients.
3. Mix well and serve.

Nutrition: Calories: 43 Total Fat: 2.5g Saturated Fat: 0.3g Cholesterol: 0mg Sodium: 22mg Carbohydrate: 4.8g Dietary Fiber: 1.2g Sugars: 2.1g Protein: 0.8g Calcium: 19mg Phosphorous: 200mg Potassium: 188mg

30. Farmer's Salad

Preparation Time: 5 minutes

Cooking Time: 5 minutes

Servings: 2 servings

INGREDIENTS:

- 60g mixed leaf salads
- 100g red pepper, diced
- 200g green beans
- 60g feta cheese
- 1 tablespoon wine vinegar
- 1 tablespoon diced onions
- Salt, pepper, sugar
- 2 tablespoons olive oil

DIRECTIONS:

1. Mix vinegar with onions, oil, and spices and mix with the salad.
2. Cut the sheep's cheese into cubes and serve with the salad. It goes well with a baguette or flatbread with herb butter.

Nutrition: Energy: 187kcal Protein: 8g Fat: 16g Carbohydrates: 4g Dietary fibers: 5g Potassium: 396mg Phosphorus: 288mg Sodium: 231mg Calcium: 188mg Phosphate: 170mg

31. Cucumber Salad

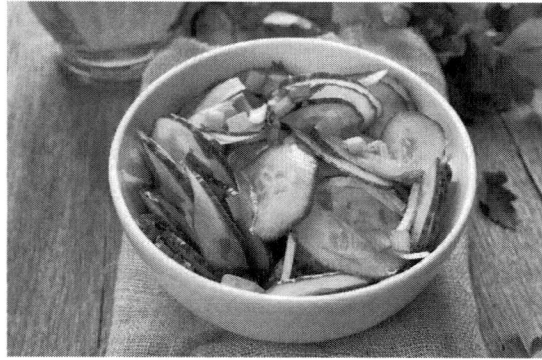

Preparation Time: 5 minutes
Cooking Time: 5 minutes
Servings: 2

INGREDIENTS:
- 1 tablespoon dried dill
- 1 onion
- ¼ cup water
- 1 cup vinegar
- 3 cucumbers
- ¾ cup white sugar

DIRECTIONS:
1. In a bowl, add all ingredients and mix well
2. Serve with dressing

Nutrition: Calories: 49 Fat: 0.1g Sodium: 341mg Potassium: 171mg Protein: 0.8g Carbohydrate: 11g Phosphorus: 24 mg

32. Barb's Asian Slaw

Preparation Time: 5 minutes
Cooking Time: 5 minutes
Servings: 2

INGREDIENTS:
- 1 cabbage head, shredded
- 4 chopped green onions
- ½ cup slivered or sliced almonds

DRESSING:
- ½ cup olive oil
- ¼ cup tamari or soy sauce
- 1 tablespoon honey or maple syrup
- 1 tablespoon baking stevia

DIRECTIONS:
1. Heat dressing ingredients in a saucepan on the stove until thoroughly mixed.
2. Mix all ingredients when you are ready to serve.

Nutrition: Calories: 205 Protein: 27g Carbohydrate: 12g Fat: 10 g Calcium 29mg, Phosphorous 76mg Potassium 27mg Sodium: 111 mg

Condiments & Seasoning

33. Basil Pesto

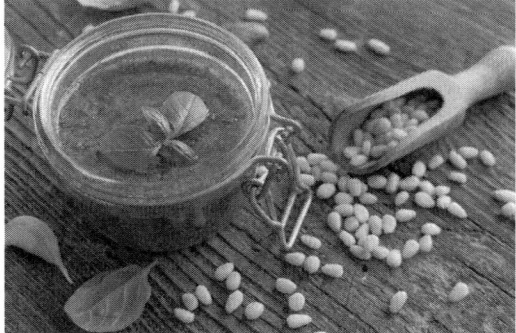

Preparation Time: 15 minutes
Cooking Time: 0 minutes
Servings: 1 ½ cups

INGREDIENTS:

- 2 cups gently packed fresh basil leaves
- 2 garlic cloves
- 2 tablespoons pine nuts
- ¼ cup olive oil
- 2 tablespoons freshly squeezed lemon juice

DIRECTIONS:

1. Pulse the basil, garlic, plus pine nuts using a food processor or blender within about 3 minutes. Drizzle the olive oil into this batter, and pulse until thick paste forms.
2. Put the lemon juice, and pulse until well blended. Store the pesto in a sealed glass container in the refrigerator for up to 2 weeks.

Nutrition: Calories: 22 Fat: 2g Sodium: 0mg Carbohydrates: 0g Phosphorus: 3mg Potassium: 10mg Protein: 0g

34. Sweet Barbecue Sauce

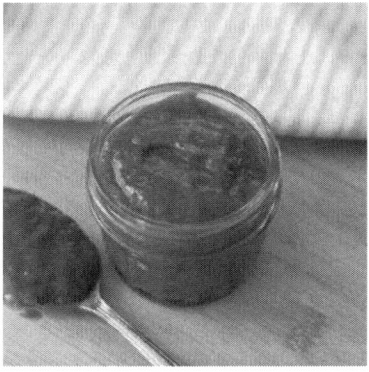

Preparation Time: 15 minutes
Cooking Time: 11 minutes
Servings: 2 cups

INGREDIENTS:

- 1 teaspoon olive oil
- ½ sweet onion, chopped
- 1 teaspoon minced garlic
- ¼ cup honey
- ¼ cup apple cider vinegar
- 2 tablespoons low-sodium tomato paste
- 1 tablespoon Dijon mustard
- 1 teaspoon hot sauce
- 1 teaspoon cornstarch

DIRECTIONS:

1. Warm-up olive oil in a medium saucepan over medium heat. Add the onion and garlic and sauté until softened, about 3 minutes.
2. Stir in ¾ cup water, the honey, vinegar, tomato paste, mustard, and hot sauce. Cook within 6 minutes.
3. In a small cup, stir together ¼ cup of water and the cornstarch. Whisk the cornstarch into the sauce and continue to cook, stirring, until the

sauce thickens about 2 minutes. Cool. Pour the sauce into a sealed glass container and store in the refrigerator for up to 1 week.

Nutrition: Calories: 14 Fat: 0g Sodium: 10mg Carbohydrates: 3g Phosphorus: 3mg Potassium: 17mg Protein: 0g

35. Low-Sodium Mayonnaise

Preparation Time: 15 minutes
Cooking Time: 0 minutes
Servings: 3

INGREDIENTS:

- 2 egg yolks
- 1 teaspoon Dijon mustard
- 1 teaspoon honey
- 2 tablespoons white vinegar
- 2 tablespoons freshly squeezed lemon juice
- 2 cups olive oil

DIRECTIONS:

1. Mix the egg yolks, mustard, honey, vinegar, and lemon juice in a large bowl. Mix in the olive oil in a thin stream. You can store this in a glass container in the refrigerator for up to 2 weeks.

Nutrition: Calories: 83 Fat: 9g Sodium: 2mg Carbohydrates: 0g Phosphorus: 2mg Potassium: 3mg Protein: 0g

36. Citrus and Mustard Marinade

Preparation Time: 15 minutes
Cooking Time: 0 minutes
Servings: ¾ cup

INGREDIENTS:

- ¼ cup freshly squeezed lemon juice
- ¼ cup freshly squeezed orange juice
- ¼ cup Dijon mustard
- 2 tablespoons honey
- 2 teaspoons chopped fresh thyme

DIRECTIONS:

1. Mix the lemon juice, orange juice, mustard, honey, and thyme until well blended in a medium bowl. Store the marinade in a sealed glass container in the refrigerator for up to 3 days. Shake before using it.

Nutrition: Calories: 35 Fat: 0g Sodium: 118mg Carbohydrates: 8g Phosphorus: 14mg Potassium: 52mg Protein: 1g

37. Fiery Honey Vinaigrette

Preparation Time: 15 minutes
Cooking Time: 0 minutes
Servings: ¾ cup

INGREDIENTS:

- 1/3 cup freshly squeezed lime juice
- ¼ cup honey
- ¼ cup olive oil
- 1 teaspoon chopped fresh basil leaves
- ½ teaspoon red pepper flakes

DIRECTIONS:

1. Mix the lime juice, honey, olive oil, basil, and red pepper flakes in a medium bowl, until well blended. Store the dressing in a glass container and store it in the fridge for up to 1 week.

Nutrition: Calories: 125 Fat: 9g Sodium: 1mg Carbohydrates: 13g Phosphorus: 1mg Potassium: 24mg Protein: 0g

38. Buttermilk Herb Dressing

Preparation Time: 15 minutes
Cooking Time: 0 minutes
Servings: 1 ½ cup

INGREDIENTS:

- ½ cup skim milk
- ½ cup Low-Sodium Mayonnaise
- 2 tablespoons apple cider vinegar
- ½ scallion, green part only, chopped
- 1 tablespoon chopped fresh dill
- 1 teaspoon chopped fresh thyme
- ½ teaspoon minced garlic
- Freshly ground black pepper

DIRECTIONS:

1. Mix the milk, mayonnaise, and vinegar until smooth in a medium bowl. Whisk in the scallion, dill, thyme, and garlic. Season with pepper. Store.

Nutrition: Calories: 31 Fat: 2g Sodium: 19mg Carbohydrates: 2g Phosphorus: 13mg Potassium: 26mg Protein: 0g

39. Poppy Seed Dressing

Preparation Time: 15 minutes
Cooking Time: 0 minutes
Servings: 2 cups

INGREDIENTS:

- ½ cup apple cider or red wine vinegar
- 1/3 cup honey
- ¼ cup freshly squeezed lemon juice
- 1 tablespoon Dijon mustard
- 1 cup olive oil
- ½ small sweet onion, minced
- 2 tablespoons poppy seeds

DIRECTIONS:

1. Mix the vinegar, honey, lemon juice, and mustard in a small bowl. Whisk in the oil, onion, and poppy seeds. Store the dressing in a sealed glass container in the refrigerator for up to 2 weeks.

Nutrition: Calories: 151 Fat: 14g Sodium: 12mg Carbohydrates: 7g Phosphorus: 13mg Potassium: 30mg Protein: 0g

40. Mediterranean Dressing

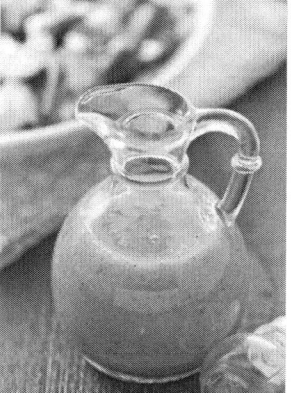

Preparation Time: 15 minutes
Cooking Time: 0 minutes
Servings: 1 cup

INGREDIENTS:

- ½ cup balsamic vinegar
- 1 teaspoon honey
- ½ teaspoon minced garlic
- 1 tablespoon dried parsley
- 1 tablespoon dried oregano
- ½ teaspoon celery seed
- Pinch freshly ground black pepper
- ½ cup olive oil

DIRECTIONS:

1. Mix the vinegar, honey, garlic, parsley, oregano, celery seed, and pepper in a small bowl. Whisk in the olive oil until emulsified. Store the dressing in a sealed glass container in the refrigerator for up to 1 week.

Nutrition: Calories: 100 Fat: 11g Sodium: 1mg Carbohydrates: 1g Phosphorus: 1mg Potassium:10mg Protein: 0g

41. Fajita Rub

Preparation Time: 15 minutes
Cooking Time: 0 minutes
Servings: ¼ cup

INGREDIENTS:

- 1½ teaspoons chili powder
- 1 teaspoon garlic powder
- 1 teaspoon roasted cumin seed
- 1 teaspoon dried oregano
- ½ teaspoon ground coriander
- ¼ teaspoon red pepper flakes

DIRECTIONS:

1. Put the chili powder, garlic powder, cumin seed, oregano, coriander, and red pepper flakes in a blender, pulse until ground and well combined. Transfer the spice mixture and store for up to 6 months.

Nutrition: Calories: 1 Fat: 0g Carbohydrates: 0g Phosphorus: 2mg Potassium: 7mg Sodium: 7mg Protein: 0g

42. Dried Herb Rub

Preparation Time: 15 minutes
Cooking Time: 0 minutes
Servings: 1/3 cup

INGREDIENTS:

- 1 tablespoon dried thyme
- 1 tablespoon dried oregano
- 1 tablespoon dried parsley
- 2 teaspoons dried basil
- 2 teaspoons ground coriander
- 2 teaspoons onion powder
- 1 teaspoon ground cumin
- 1 teaspoon garlic powder
- 1 teaspoon paprika
- ½ teaspoon cayenne pepper

DIRECTIONS:

1. Put the thyme, oregano, parsley, basil, coriander, onion powder, cumin, garlic powder, paprika, and cayenne pepper in a blender, and pulse until the ingredients are ground and well combined. Transfer the rub to a small container with a lid. Store in a cool, dry area for up to 6 months.

Nutrition: Calories: 3 Fat: 0g Carbohydrates: 1g Phosphorus: 3mg Potassium: 16mg Sodium: 1mg Protein: 0g

43. Mediterranean Seasoning

Preparation Time: 15 minutes
Cooking Time: 0 minutes
Servings: 1

INGREDIENTS:

- 2 tablespoons dried oregano
- 1 tablespoon dried thyme
- 2 teaspoons dried rosemary, chopped finely or crushed

- 2 teaspoons dried basil
- 1 teaspoon dried marjoram
- 1 teaspoon dried parsley flakes

DIRECTIONS:

1. Mix the oregano, thyme, rosemary, basil, marjoram, and parsley in a small bowl until well combined. Transfer then store.

Nutrition: Calories: 1 Fat: 0g Carbohydrates: 0g Phosphorus: 1mg Potassium: 6mg Sodium: 0mg Protein: 0g

44. Hot Curry Powder

Preparation Time: 15 minutes
Cooking Time: 0 minutes
Servings: 1 ¼ cup

INGREDIENTS:

- ¼ cup ground cumin
- ¼ cup ground coriander
- 3 tablespoons turmeric
- 2 tablespoons sweet paprika
- 2 tablespoons ground mustard
- 1 tablespoon fennel powder
- ½ teaspoon green chili powder
- 2 teaspoons ground cardamom
- 1 teaspoon ground cinnamon
- ½ teaspoon ground cloves

DIRECTIONS:

1. Pulse the cumin, coriander, turmeric, paprika, mustard, fennel powder, green chili powder, cardamom, cinnamon, plus cloves using a blender, until the fixing is ground and well combined. Transfer it to a small container, put in a cool, dry place for up to 6 months.

Nutrition: Calories: 19 Fat: 1g Carbohydrates: 3g Phosphorus: 24mg Potassium: 93mg Sodium: 5mg Protein: 1g

45. Cajun Seasoning

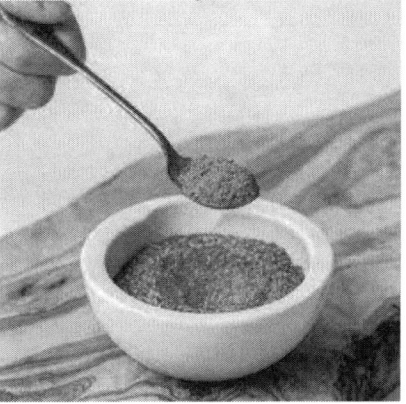

Preparation Time: 15 minutes
Cooking Time: 0 minutes
Servings: 1 ¼ cup

INGREDIENTS:

- ½ cup sweet paprika
- ¼ cup garlic powder
- 3 tablespoons onion powder
- 3 tablespoons freshly ground black pepper
- 2 tablespoons dried oregano
- 1 tablespoon cayenne pepper
- 1 tablespoon dried thyme

DIRECTIONS:

1. Pulse the paprika, garlic powder, onion powder, black pepper, oregano, cayenne pepper, and thyme in a blender until the fixing is ground and well combined.

Nutrition: Calories: 7 Fat: 0g Carbohydrates: 2g Phosphorus: 8mg Potassium: 40mg Sodium: 1mg Protein: 0g

46. Apple Pie Spice

Preparation Time: 15 minutes
Cooking Time: 0 minutes
Servings: 1/3 cup

INGREDIENTS:

- ¼ cup ground cinnamon
- 2 teaspoons ground nutmeg
- 2 teaspoons ground ginger
- 1 teaspoon allspice
- ½ teaspoon ground cloves

DIRECTIONS:

1. Mix the cinnamon, nutmeg, ginger, allspice, and cloves in a small bowl. Store for up to 6 months.

Nutrition: Calories: 6 Fat: 0g Carbohydrates: 1g Phosphorus: 2mg Potassium: 12mg Sodium: 1mg Protein: 0g

47. Ras El Hanout

Preparation Time: 5 minutes
Cooking Time: 0 minutes
Servings: ½ cup

INGREDIENTS:

- 2 teaspoons ground nutmeg
- 2 teaspoons ground coriander
- 2 teaspoons ground cumin
- 2 teaspoons turmeric
- 2 teaspoons cinnamon
- 1 teaspoon cardamom
- 1 teaspoon sweet paprika
- 1 teaspoon ground mace
- 1 teaspoon freshly ground black pepper
- 1 teaspoon cayenne pepper
- ½ teaspoon ground allspice
- ½ teaspoon ground cloves

DIRECTIONS:

1. Mix the nutmeg, coriander, cumin, turmeric, cinnamon, cardamom, paprika, mace, black pepper, cayenne pepper, allspice, and cloves in a small bowl. Store.

Nutrition: Calories: 5 Fat: 0g Carbohydrates: 1g Phosphorus: 3mg Potassium: 17mg Sodium: 1mg Protein: 0g

48. Poultry Seasoning

Preparation Time: 15 minutes
Cooking Time: 0 minutes
Servings: ½ cup

INGREDIENTS:

- 2 tablespoons ground thyme
- 2 tablespoons ground marjoram
- 1 tablespoon ground sage
- 1 tablespoon ground celery seed
- 1 teaspoon ground rosemary
- 1 teaspoon freshly ground black pepper

DIRECTIONS:

1. Mix the thyme, marjoram, sage, celery seed, rosemary, and pepper in a small bowl. Store for up to 6 months.

Nutrition: Calories: 3 Fat: 0g Carbohydrates: 0g Phosphorus: 3mg Potassium: 10mg Sodium: 1mg Protein: 0g

49. Berbere Spice Mix

Preparation Time: 15 minutes
Cooking Time: 4 minutes
Servings: ½ cup

INGREDIENTS:

- 1 tablespoon coriander seeds
- 1 teaspoon cumin seeds
- 1 teaspoon fenugreek seeds
- ¼ teaspoon black peppercorns
- ¼ teaspoon whole allspice berries
- 4 whole cloves
- 4 dried chilis, stemmed and seeded
- ¼ cup dried onion flakes
- 2 tablespoons ground cardamom
- 1 tablespoon sweet paprika
- 1 teaspoon ground ginger
- ½ teaspoon ground nutmeg
- ½ teaspoon ground cinnamon

DIRECTIONS:

1. Put the coriander, cumin, fenugreek, peppercorns, allspice, and cloves in a small skillet over medium heat. Lightly toast the spices, swirling the skillet frequently, for about 4 minutes or until the spices are fragrant.
2. Remove the skillet, then let the spices cool for about 10 minutes. Transfer the toasted spices to a blender with the chilis and onion, and grind until the mixture is finely ground.
3. Transfer the ground spice mixture to a small bowl and stir together the cardamom, paprika, ginger, nutmeg, and cinnamon until thoroughly combined. Store the spice mixture in a small container with a lid for up to 6 months.

Nutrition: Calories: 8 Fat: 0g Carbohydrates: 2g Phosphorus: 7mg Potassium: 37mg Sodium: 14mg Protein: 0g

Snack and Appetizer

50. Easy No-Bake Coconut Cookies

Preparation Time: 5 minutes
Cooking Time: 10 minutes
Servings: 2

INGREDIENTS:

- 3 cups finely shredded coconut flakes
- 1 cup melted coconut oil
- 1 teaspoon liquid stevia

DIRECTIONS:

1. Prepare all ingredients in a large bowl; stir until well blended.
2. Form the mixture into small balls and arrange them on a paper-lined baking tray.
3. Press each cookie down with a fork and refrigerate until firm. Enjoy!

Nutrition: Calories: 99 Fat: 10 g Carbohydrate: 2 g Protein: 3 g Sodium: 7 mg Potassium: 105mg Phosphorus: 11mg

51. Roasted Chili-Vinegar Peanuts

Preparation Time: 5 minutes
Cooking Time: 10 minutes
Servings: 2

INGREDIENTS:

- 1 tablespoon coconut oil
- 2 cups raw peanuts, unsalted
- 2 teaspoon sea salt
- 2 tablespoon apple cider vinegar
- 1 teaspoon chili powder
- 1 teaspoon fresh lime zest

DIRECTIONS:

1. Preheat oven to 350°F.
2. In a large bowl, toss together coconut oil, peanuts, and salt until well coated.
3. Transfer to a rimmed baking sheet and roast in the oven for about 15 minutes or until fragrant.
4. Transfer the roasted peanuts to a bowl and add vinegar, chili powder, and lime zest.
5. Toss to coat well and serve.

Nutrition: Calories: 447 Fat: 39.5g Carbohydrate: 12.3 g Protein: 18.9 g Sodium: 160 mg Potassium: 200mg Phosphorus: 0mg

52. Veggie Snack

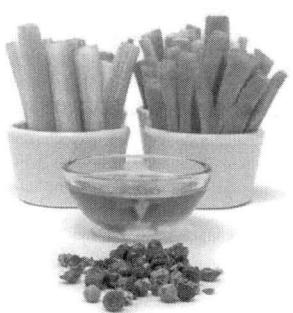

Preparation Time: 5 minutes
Cooking Time: 10 minutes
Servings: 2

INGREDIENTS:

- 1 large yellow pepper
- 5 carrots
- 5 stalks celery

DIRECTIONS:

1. Clean the carrots and rinse them under running water.
2. Rinse celery and yellow pepper. Remove seeds of pepper and chop the veggies into small sticks.
3. Put in a bowl and serve.

Nutrition: Calories: 189 Fat: 0.5 g Carbohydrate: 44.3 g Protein: 5 g Sodium: 282 mg Potassium: 0mg Phosphorus: 0mg

53. Healthy Spiced Nuts

Preparation Time: 10 minutes
Cooking Time: 10 minutes
Servings: 4

INGREDIENTS:

- 1 tablespoon extra-virgin olive oil
- ¼ cup walnuts
- ¼ cup pecans
- ¼ cup almonds
- ½ teaspoon sea salt
- ½ teaspoon cumin
- ½ teaspoon pepper
- 1 teaspoon chili powder

DIRECTIONS:

1. Put the skillet on medium heat and toast the nuts until lightly browned.
2. Prepare the spice mixture and add black pepper, cumin, chili, and salt.
3. Put extra virgin olive oil and sprinkle with spice mixture to the toasted nuts before serving.

Nutrition: Calories: 88 Fat: 8g Carbohydrate: 4g Protein: 2.5g Sodium: 51mg Potassium: 88mg Phosphorus: 6.3mg

54. Roasted Asparagus

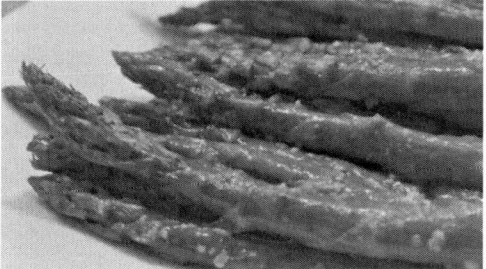

Preparation Time: 5 minutes
Cooking Time: 10 minutes
Servings: 4

INGREDIENTS:

- 1 tablespoon extra-virgin olive oil
- 1-pound fresh asparagus
- 1 medium lemon, zested
- 1/2 teaspoon freshly grated nutmeg
- 1/2 teaspoon kosher salt
- ½ teaspoon black pepper

DIRECTIONS:

1. Preheat your oven to 500°F.
2. Put asparagus on an aluminum foil and add extra virgin olive oil.
3. Prepare asparagus in a single layer and fold the edges of the foil.
4. Cook in the oven for 5 minutes. Continue roasting until browned.
5. Add the roasted asparagus with nutmeg, salt, zest, and pepper before serving.

Nutrition: Calories: 55 Fat: 3.8 g Carbohydrate: 4.7 g Protein: 2.5 g Sodium: 98mg Potassium: 172mg Phosphorus: 35mg

55. Low-Fat Mango Salsa

Preparation Time: 10 minutes
Cooking Time: 10 minutes
Servings: 4

INGREDIENTS:

- 1 cup cucumber, chopped
- 2 cups mango, diced
- ½ cup cilantro, minced
- 2 tablespoons fresh lime juice
- 1 tablespoon scallions, minced
- ¼ teaspoon chipotle powder
- ¼ teaspoon sea salt

DIRECTIONS:

1. Mix the ingredients in a bowl and serve or refrigerate.

Nutrition: Calories: 155 Fat: 0.6 g Carbohydrate: 38.2 g Protein: 1.4 g Sodium: 3.2 mg Potassium: 221mg Phosphorus: 27mg

56. Carrot and Parsnips French Fries

Preparation Time: 15 minutes
Cooking Time: 20 minutes
Servings: 2

INGREDIENTS:

- 6 large carrots
- 6 large parsnips
- 2 tablespoons extra virgin olive oil
- ½ teaspoon of sea salt

DIRECTIONS:

1. Chop the carrots and parsnips into 2-inch slices and then cut each into thin sticks.
2. Toss together the carrots and parsnip sticks with extra virgin olive oil and salt in a bowl and spread into a baking sheet lined with parchment paper.
3. Bake the sticks at 425°F for about 20 minutes or until browned.

Nutrition: Calories: 179 Fat: 4g Carbohydrate: 14g Protein: 11g Sodium: 27.3mg Potassium: 625mg Phosphorus: 116mg

57. Apple & Strawberry Snack

Preparation Time: 5 minutes
Cooking Time: 2 minutes
Servings: 2

INGREDIENTS:

- ½ apple, cored and sliced
- 2-3 strawberries
- dash of ground cinnamon
- 2-3 drops stevia 2-3 drops

DIRECTIONS:

1. In a bowl, mix strawberries and apples and sprinkle with stevia and cinnamon.
2. Microwave for about 1-2 minutes. Serve warm.

Nutrition: Calories: 145 Fat: 0.8 g Carbohydrate: 34.2 g Protein: 1.6 g Sodium: 20 mg Potassium: 0mg Phosphorus: 0mg

58. Candied Macadamia Nuts

Preparation Time: 5 minutes
Cooking Time: 15 minutes
Servings: 2

INGREDIENTS:

- 2 cups macadamia nuts
- 1 tablespoon extra-virgin olive oil
- 2 tablespoons honey

DIRECTIONS:

1. Toss ingredients in a bowl and spread into a baking dish.
2. Bake for 15 minutes at 350°F.
3. Let cool before serving.

Nutrition: Calories: 200 Fat: 18 g Carbohydrate: 10g Protein: 1g Sodium: 5 mg Potassium: 55mg Phosphorus: 10mg

59. Baba Ghanouj

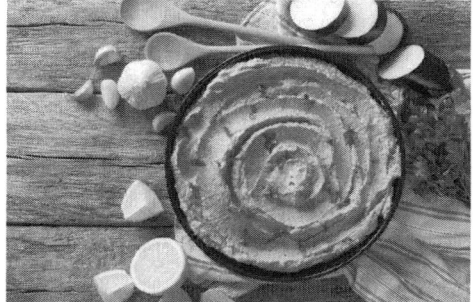

Preparation Time: 10 minutes
Cooking Time: 1 hour and 20 minutes
Servings: 2

INGREDIENTS:

- 1 large aubergine, cut in half lengthwise
- 1 head of garlic, unpeeled
- 30 ml (2 tablespoons) of olive oil
- Lemon juice to taste

DIRECTIONS:

1. Preheat the oven to 350°F.
2. Place the eggplant on the plate, skin side up. Roast until the meat is very tender and detaches easily from the skin, about 1 hour depending on the eggplant's size. Let cool.
3. Meanwhile, cut the tip of the garlic cloves. Put garlic cloves in a square aluminum foil. Fold the edges of the sheet and fold together to form a tightly wrapped foil.
4. Roast with the eggplant until tender, about 20 minutes. Let cool. Purée the pods with a garlic press.
5. With a spoon, scoop out the eggplant's flesh and place it in the bowl of a food processor. Add the garlic puree, the oil, and the lemon juice. Stir until purée is smooth and pepper.
6. Serve with mini pita bread.

Nutrition: Calories: 110 Fat: 12g Carbohydrate: 5g Protein: 1g Sodium: 180mg Potassium: 207mg Phosphorus: 81mg

60. Herbal Cream Cheese Tartines

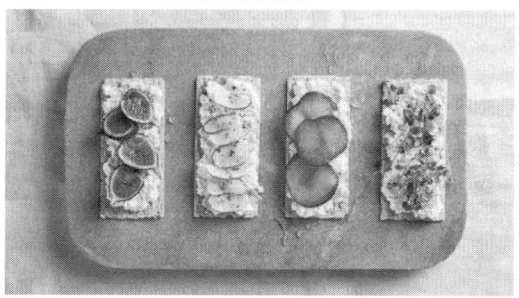

Preparation Time: 15 minutes
Cooking Time: 15 minutes
Servings: 2

INGREDIENTS:

- 1 clove garlic, halved
- 1 cup cream cheese spread
- ¼ cup chopped herbs such as chives, dill, parsley, tarragon, or thyme
- 2 tablespoons minced French shallot or onion
- ½ teaspoon black pepper

- 2 tablespoons water

DIRECTIONS:

1. Combine the cream cheese, herbs, shallot, pepper, and water in a medium-sized bowl with a hand blender.
2. Serve the cream cheese with the rusks.

Nutrition: Calories: 476 Fat: 9g Carbohydrate: 75g Protein: 23g Sodium: 885mg Potassium: 312mg Phosphorus: 165mg

61. Spicy Crab Dip

Preparation Time: 10 minutes
Cooking Time: 20 minutes
Servings: 2

INGREDIENTS:

- 1 can of 8 oz. softened cream cheese
- 1 tbsp. finely chopped onions
- 1 tbsp. lemon juice
- 2 tbsp. Worcestershire sauce
- 1/8 tsp. black pepper Cayenne pepper to taste
- 2 tbsp. to s. of almond milk or non-fortified rice drink
- 1 can of 6 oz. of crabmeat

DIRECTIONS:

1. Preheat the oven to 375°F.
2. Pour the cheese cream into a bowl. Add the onions, lemon juice, Worcestershire sauce, black pepper, and cayenne pepper. Mix well. Stir in the almond milk/rice drink.
3. Add the crabmeat and mix until you obtain a homogeneous mixture.
4. Pour the mixture into a baking dish. Cook without covering for 15 minutes or until bubbles appear. Serve hot with triangle cut pita bread.
5. Microwave until bubbles appear, about 4 minutes, stirring every 1 to 2 minutes.

Nutrition: Calories: 42 Fat: 0.5g Carbohydrate: 2g Protein: 7g Sodium: 167mg Potassium: 130mg Phosphorus: 139mg

62. Blueberry-Ricotta Swirl

Preparation Time: 5 minutes
Cooking Time: 5 minutes
Servings: 2

INGREDIENTS:

- ½ cup fresh or frozen blueberries
- ½ cup part-skim ricotta cheese
- 1 teaspoon sugar
- ½ teaspoon lemon zest (optional)

DIRECTIONS:

1. If using frozen blueberries, warm them in a saucepan over medium heat until they are thawed but not hot.
2. Meanwhile, mix the sugar with the ricotta in a medium bowl.
3. Mix the blueberries into the ricotta, leaving a few out. Taste, and add more sugar if desired. Top with the remaining blueberries and lemon zest (if using).

Nutrition: Calories: 113 Total Fat: 5g Saturated Fat: 3g Cholesterol: 19mg Sodium: 62mg Carbohydrates: 10g Fiber: 1g Added Sugars: 2g

Protein: 7g Potassium: 98mg Phosphorus 64mg Vitamin K: 7mcg

63. Cranberry Cabbage

Preparation Time: 10 minutes
Cooking Time: 20 minutes
Servings: 8

INGREDIENTS:

- 10 ounces canned whole-berry cranberry sauce
- 1 tablespoon fresh lemon juice
- 1 medium head red cabbage
- 1/4 teaspoon ground cloves

DIRECTIONS:

1. Place the cranberry sauce, lemon juice, and cloves in a large pan and bring to a boil.
2. Add the cabbage and reduce it to a simmer.
3. Cook until the cabbage is tender, occasionally stirring to make sure the sauce does not stick.
4. Delicious served with beef, lamb, or pork.

Nutrition: Calories: 73 Fat: 0g Carbohydrate: 18g Protein: 1g Sodium: 32mg Potassium: 138mg Phosphorous: 18mg

64. Carrot-Apple Casserole

Preparation Time: 15 minutes
Cooking Time: 50 minutes
Servings: 8

INGREDIENTS:

- 6 large carrots, peeled and sliced
- 4 large apples, peeled and sliced
- 3 tablespoons butter
- ½ cup apple juice
- 5 tablespoons all-purpose flour
- 2 tablespoons brown sugar
- ½ teaspoon ground nutmeg

DIRECTIONS:

1. Preheat oven to 350° F.
2. Let the carrots boil for 5 minutes or until tender. Drain.
3. Arrange the carrots and apples in a large casserole dish.
4. Put and mix well the flour, brown sugar, and nutmeg in a small bowl.
5. Rub in butter to make a crumb topping.
6. Sprinkle the crumb over the carrots and apples, then drizzle with juice.
7. Bake until bubbling and golden brown.

Nutrition: Calories: 245 Fat: 6g Carbohydrate: 49g Protein: 1g Sodium: 91mg Potassium: 169mg Phosphorous: 17mg

65. Garlic Mashed Potatoes

Preparation Time: 5 minutes
Cooking Time: 20 minutes
Servings: 4

INGREDIENTS:

- 2 medium potatoes, peeled and sliced
- ¼ cup butter
- ¼ cup 1% low-fat milk
- 2 garlic cloves

DIRECTIONS:

1. Double-boil or soak the potatoes to reduce potassium if you are on a low potassium diet.

2. Boil potatoes and garlic until soft. Drain.
3. Beat the potatoes and garlic with butter and milk until smooth.

Nutrition: Calories: 168 Carbohydrate: 29g Protein: 5g Sodium: 59 Potassium: 161g Phosphorous: 57mg

Soups & Stews

66. Chicken Noodle Soup

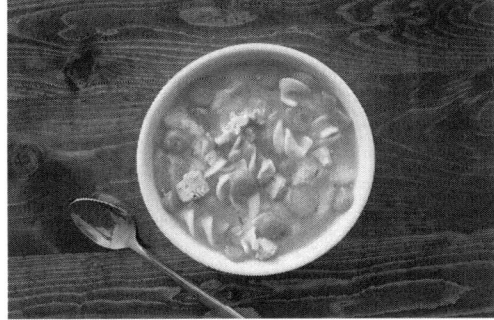

Preparation Time: 10 minutes
Cooking Time: 25 minutes
Servings: 2

INGREDIENTS:

- 1 1/2 cups low-sodium vegetable broth
- 1 cup water
- 1/4 tsp poultry seasoning
- 1/4 tsp black pepper
- 1 cup chicken strips
- 1/4 cup carrot
- 2 oz egg noodles, uncooked

DIRECTIONS:

1. Toss all the ingredients into a slow cooker
2. Cook soup on high heat for 25 minutes.
3. Serve warm.

Nutrition: Calories: 103 Protein: 8 g Carbohydrates: 11 g Fat: 3 g Cholesterol: 4 mg Sodium: 355 mg Potassium: 264 mg Phosphorus: 128 mg Calcium: 46 mg Fiber: 4.0 g

67. Classic Chicken Soup

Preparation Time: 5-10 minutes
Cooking Time: 35 minutes
Serving: 2

INGREDINETS:

- 2 teaspoons minced garlic
- 2 celery stalks, chopped
- 1 tablespoon unsalted butter
- ½ sweet onion, diced
- 1 carrot, diced
- 4 cups water
- 1 teaspoon chopped fresh thyme
- 2 cups chopped cooked chicken breast
- 1 cup chicken stock
- Black pepper (ground), to taste
- 2 tablespoons chopped fresh parsley

DIRECTIONS:

1. Take a medium-large cooking pot, heat oil over medium heat.
2. Add onion and stir-cook until it becomes translucent and softened.
3. Add garlic and stir-cook until it becomes fragrant.
4. Add celery, carrot, chicken, chicken stock, and water.
5. Boil the mixture.
6. Over low heat, simmer the mixture for about 25-30 minutes until veggies are tender.
7. Mix in thyme and cook for 2 minutes. Season to taste with black pepper.
8. Serve warm with parsley on top.

Nutrition: Calories: 135 Fat: 6g Phosphorus: 122mg Potassium: 208mg Sodium: 74mg Carbohydrates: 3g Protein: 15g.

68. Beef Okra Soup

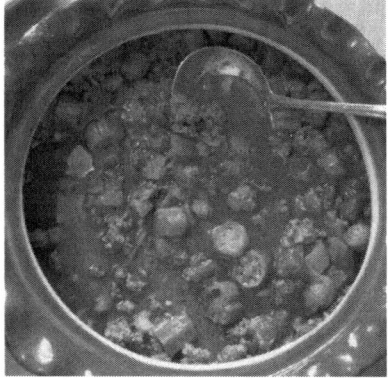

Preparation Time: 10 minutes
Cooking Time: 45-55 minutes
Serving: 2

INGREDIENTS:

- ½ cup okra
- ½ teaspoon basil
- ½ cup carrots, diced
- 3 ½ cups water
- 1-pound beef stew meat
- 1 cup raw sliced onions
- ½ cup green peas
- 1 teaspoon black pepper
- ½ teaspoon thyme
- ½ cup corn kernels

DIRECTIONS:

1. Take a medium-large cooking pot, heat oil over medium heat.
2. Add water, beef stew meat, black pepper, onions, basil, thyme, and stir-cook for 40-45 minutes until meat is tender.
3. Add all veggies. Over low heat, simmer the mixture for about 20-25 minutes. Add more water if needed.
4. Serve soup warm.

Nutrition: Calories: 187 Fat: 12g Phosphorus: 119mg Potassium: 288mg Sodium: 59mg Carbohydrates: 7g Protein: 11g

69. Chicken Pasta Soup

Preparation Time: 10 minutes
Cooking Time: 20 minutes
Serving: 2

INGREDIENTS:

- 1 ½ cups baby spinach
- 2 tablespoons orzo (tiny pasta)
- 1 tablespoon dry white wine
- 1 14-ounce low sodium chicken broth
- 2 plum tomatoes, chopped
- ½ teaspoon Italian seasoning
- 1 large shallot, chopped
- 1 small zucchini, diced
- 8-ounces chicken tenders
- 1 tablespoon extra-virgin olive oil

DIRECTIONS:

1. Take a medium saucepan or skillet, add oil. Heat over medium heat.
2. Add chicken and stir-cook for 3 minutes until evenly brown. Set aside.
3. In the pan, add zucchini, Italian seasoning, shallot; stir-cook until veggies are softened.
4. Add tomatoes, wine, broth, and orzo.
5. Boil the mixture.
6. Over low heat, cover, and simmer the mixture for about 3 minutes.
7. Mix in spinach and cooked chicken; stir and serve warm.

Nutrition: Calories: 103 Fat: 3g Phosphorus: 125m Potassium: 264mg Sodium: 84mg Carbohydrates: 6g Protein: 12g.

70. Cabbage Turkey Soup

Preparation Time: 10 minutes
Cooking Time: 40-45 minutes
Serving: 2

INGREDIENTS:

- ½ cup shredded green cabbage
- ½ cup bulgur
- 2 dried bay leaves
- 2 tablespoons chopped fresh parsley
- 1 teaspoon chopped fresh sage
- 1 teaspoon chopped fresh thyme
- 1 celery stalk, chopped
- 1 carrot, sliced thin
- ½ sweet onion, chopped
- 1 teaspoon minced garlic
- 1 teaspoon olive oil
- ½ pound cooked ground turkey, 93% lean
- 4 cups water
- 1 cup chicken stock
- Pinch red pepper flakes
- Black pepper (ground), to taste

DIRECTIONS:

1. Take a large saucepan or cooking pot, add oil. Heat over medium heat.
2. Add turkey and stir-cook for 4-5 minutes until evenly brown.
3. Add onion and garlic and sauté for about 3 minutes to soften veggies.
4. Add water, chicken stock, cabbage, bulgur, celery, carrot, and bay leaves.
5. Boil the mixture.
6. Over low heat, cover, and simmer the mixture for about 30-35 minutes until bulgur is cooked well and tender.
7. Remove bay leaves. Add parsley, sage, thyme, and red pepper flakes; stir mixture and season with black pepper. Serve warm.

Nutrition: Calories: 83 Fat: 4g Phosphorus: 91mg Potassium: 185mg Sodium: 63mg Carbohydrates: 2g Protein: 8g.

71. Chicken Fajita Soup

Preparation Time: 10 minutes
Cooking Time: 6 hours 30 minutes
Servings: 2

INGREDIENTS:

- 2 pounds of boneless skinless chicken breasts
- 1 onion chopped
- 1 green pepper chopped
- 3 garlic cloves minced
- 1 tablespoon butter
- 6 ounces cream cheese
- salt and pepper to taste

DIRECTIONS:

1. Add boneless skinless chicken breasts to a slow cooker and cook for 3 hours on high or 6 hours on low in a cup of chicken broth. Season with salt and pepper.
2. When the chicken is done, remove from the slow cooker and shred. (You can strain the leftover broth for the soup.)
3. In a large saucepan fry green pepper, onion, and garlic in 1 tablespoon of butter until they are translucent (2 to 3 minutes). Mash the cream cheese into the veggies with a spoon so that it will combine smoothly as it melts.

Nutrition: Calories: 306kcal Carbohydrates: 8.2g Protein: 26g Fat: 17g Saturated Fat: 9g Cholesterol: 120mg; Sodium: 880mg Potassium: 757mg Fiber: 1.6g; Sugar: 3g

72. Cream of Chicken Soup

Preparation Time: 10 minutes
Cooking Time: 20 minutes
Servings: 2

INGREDIENTS:

- 2 cups cauliflower florets
- 2/3 cup unsweetened original almond milk
- 1 cup chicken broth
- 1 teaspoon onion powder
- ½ teaspoon grey sea salt
- ¼ teaspoon garlic powder
- ¼ teaspoon freshly ground black pepper
- 1/8 teaspoon celery seed (optional)
- 1/8 teaspoon dried thyme
- ¼ cup Beef Gelatin

DIRECTIONS:

1. Place all ingredients, except cooked chicken and gelatin, in a small saucepan. Cover and bring to a boil over medium heat. Turn heat to low and cook for about 7 to 8 minutes, until cauliflower is softened. Remove from the heat. Add around ½ cup of the hot liquid to a medium-sized bowl using a ladle. Add gelatin, one scoop at a time. Stir until dissolved, then add the next scoop.
2. Serve immediately.

Nutrition: Calories: 198 Calories from Fat: 62.1 Total Fat: 6.9 g Saturated Fat: 1.1 g Cholesterol: 24 mg Sodium: 672 mg Phosphorus: 36m Potassium: 194mg Carbs: 9.4 g Dietary Fiber: 3.8 g Net Carbs: 5.6 g Sugars: 3.3 g Protein: 26.4 g.

73. Turkey & Lemon-Grass Soup

Preparation Time: 5 minutes
Cooking Time: 40 minutes
Serving: 2

INGREDIENTS:

1. 1 fresh lime
2. ¼ cup fresh basil leaves
3. 1 tablespoon cilantro
4. 1 cup canned and drained water chestnuts
5. 1 tablespoon coconut oil
6. 1 thumb-size minced ginger piece
7. 2 chopped scallions
8. 1 finely chopped green chili
9. 4 oz. skinless and sliced turkey breasts
10. 1 minced garlic clove
11. ½ finely sliced stick lemongrass
12. 1 chopped white onion
13. 4 cups water

DIRECTIONS:

1. Crush the lemongrass, cilantro, chili, 1 tablespoon oil, and basil leaves in a blender or with the help of a pestle and mortar, to form a paste. Keep it aside.
2. Heat a large pan/wok with 1 tablespoon olive oil on high heat.
3. Sauté the onions, garlic, and ginger until soft.
4. Add the turkey and brown each side for 4-5 minutes.

5. Add the broth and stir.
6. Now add the prepared paste and stir.
7. Next, add the water chestnuts, turn down the heat slightly and allow it to simmer for 25-30 minutes or until turkey is thoroughly cooked through.
8. Serve hot with the green onion sprinkled over the top.

Nutrition: Calories: 123 Protein: 10 g Carbohydrate: 12 g Fat: 3 g Sodium: 501 mg Potassium: 151 mg Phosphorus: 110 mg.

74. Paprika Pork Soup

Preparation Time: 5 minutes
Cooking Time: 35 minutes
Servings: 2

INGREDIENTS:

- 4 oz. sliced pork loin
- 1 teaspoon black pepper
- 2 minced garlic cloves
- 1 cup baby spinach
- 3 cups water
- 1 tablespoon extra-virgin olive oil
- 1 chopped onion
- 1 tablespoon paprika

DIRECTIONS:

1. In a large pot, add the oil, chopped onion and minced garlic.
2. Sauté for 5 minutes on low heat.
3. Add the pork slices to the onions and cook for 7-8 minutes or until browned.
4. Stir in the spinach, reduce heat and simmer for a further 20 minutes or until pork is thoroughly cooked through.
5. Season with pepper to serve.

Nutrition: Calories: 165 Protein: 13 g Carbohydrate: 10 g Fat: 9g Sodium: 269 mg Potassium: 486 mg Phosphorus: 158 mg

75. White Fish Stew

Preparation Time: 10 minutes
Cooking Time: 35 minutes
Servings: 2

INGREDIENTS:

- 4 white fish fillets
- 1 cup of water
- 1 onion, sliced
- 1/2 teaspoon paprika
- 1/4 cup olive oil
- 1/4 teaspoon pepper
- 1 teaspoon salt

DIRECTIONS:

1. Add olive oil, paprika, onion, water, pepper, and salt into the saucepan. Stir well and bring to boil over medium-high heat.
2. Turn heat to medium-low and simmer for 15 minutes.
3. Add white fish fillets and cook until fish is cooked.
4. Serve and enjoy.

Nutrition: Calories: 513 Fat: 32.3 g Carbohydrates: 3.7 g Sugar: 1.6 g Protein: 50.7 g Cholesterol: 158 mg Phosphorus: 120mg Potassium: 117mg Sodium: 75mg

76. Pumpkin, Coconut and Sage Soup

Preparation Time: 10 minutes
Cooking Time: 30 minutes
Servings: 2

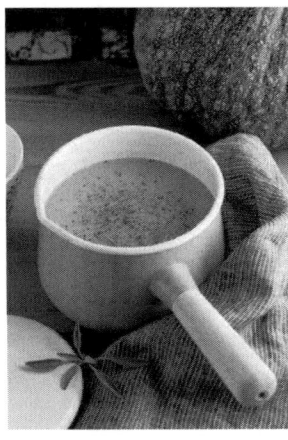

INGREDIENTS:

- 1 cup pumpkin, canned
- 6 cups chicken broth
- 1 cup low-fat coconut almond milk
- 1 teaspoon sage, chopped
- 3 garlic cloves, peeled
- Sunflower seeds and pepper to taste

DIRECTIONS:

1. Take a stockpot and add all the ingredients except coconut almond milk into it.
2. Place stockpot over medium heat.
3. Let it bring to a boil.
4. Reduce heat to simmer for 30 minutes.
5. Add the coconut almond milk and stir.
6. Serve bacon and enjoy!

Nutrition: Calories: 145 Fat: 12g Carbohydrates: 8g Protein: 6g Phosphorus: 110mg Potassium: 117mg Sodium: 75mg

77. The Kale and Green Lettuce Soup

Preparation Time: 5 minutes
Cooking Time: 10 minutes
Servings: 2

INGREDIENTS:

- 3 ounces coconut oil
- 8 ounces kale, chopped
- 4 1/3 cups coconut almond milk
- Pepper to taste

DIRECTIONS:

1. Take a skillet and place it over medium heat.
2. Add kale and sauté for 2-3 minutes
3. Add kale to blender.
4. Add water, pepper, coconut almond milk to the blender as well.
5. Blend until smooth and pour mix into bowl.
6. Serve and enjoy!

Nutrition: Calories: 124 Fat: 13g Carbohydrates: 7g Protein: 4.2g Phosphorus: 110mg Potassium: 117mg Sodium: 105mg

78. Sweet Potato and Corn Soup

Preparation Time: 10 minutes
Cooking Time: 20 minutes
Servings: 2

INGREDIENTS:

- ¼ cup extra-virgin olive oil or coconut oil
- 1 medium zucchini, cut into ¼-inch dice
- 1 cup broccoli florets
- 1 cup thinly sliced mushrooms
- 1 small onion, cut into ¼-inch dice
- 4 cups vegetable broth
- 2 cups peeled carrots cut into ¼-inch dice
- 1 cup frozen corn kernels
- 1 cup coconut almond milk or almond milk

- 2 tablespoons finely chopped fresh flat-leaf parsley
- 1 teaspoon salt
- ¼ teaspoon freshly ground black pepper

DIRECTIONS:

1. In a huge pot, heat the oil on high heat.
2. Add the zucchini, broccoli, mushrooms, and onion and sauté until softened, 5 to 8 minutes.
3. Pour the broth and carrots and place it to a boil.
4. Reduce the heat to a simmer and cook until the carrots are tender, 5 to 7 minutes.
5. Add the corn, coconut almond milk, parsley, salt, and pepper. Cook on low heat up to the corn is heated through and serve.

Nutrition: Calories: 402 Fat: 29g Carbohydrates: 31gSugar: 9gFiber: 6g Protein: 10g Sodium: 1406mg

79. Chickpea Curry Soup

Preparation Time: 10 minutes
Cooking Time: 25 minutes
Servings: 2

INGREDIENTS:

- ¼ cup extra-virgin olive oil or coconut oil
- 1 medium onion, finely chopped
- 2 garlic cloves, sliced
- 1 large apple, cored, peeled, and cut into ¼-inch dice
- 2 teaspoons curry powder
- 1 teaspoon salt
- 3 cups peeled butternut squash cut into ½-inch dice
- 3 cups vegetable broth
- 1 cup full-fat coconut almond milk
- 1 (15-ounce) can chickpeas, drained and rinsed
- 2 tablespoons finely chopped fresh cilantro

DIRECTIONS:

1. In a huge pot, heat the oil on high heat.
2. Add the onion and garlic and sauté until the onion begins to brown, 6 to 8 minutes.
3. Put the apple, curry powder, and salt and sauté to toast the curry powder, 1 to 2 minutes.
4. Put the squash and broth then bring to a boil.
5. Lower the heat then cook until the squash is tender about 10 minutes.
6. Stir in the coconut almond milk.
7. Using an immersion blender, purée the soup in the pot until smooth.
8. Stir in the chickpeas and cilantro, heat through for 1 to 2 minutes, and serve.

Nutrition: Calories: 469 Fat: 30g Carbohydrates: 45g Sugar: 14g Fiber: 10gProtein: 12gSodium: 1174mg

80. Onion, Kale and White Bean Soup

Preparation Time: 15 minutes
Cooking Time: 25 minutes
Servings: 2

INGREDIENTS:

- ¼ cup extra-virgin olive oil
- 1 large onion, thinly sliced
- 2 garlic cloves, thinly sliced
- 1 teaspoon salt
- ¼ teaspoon freshly ground black pepper
- 1/8 Teaspoon red pepper flakes (optional)
- 3 cups stemmed kale leaves cut into ½-inch pieces
- 4 cups vegetable broth
- 1 (15½-ounce) can white beans, drained and rinsed
- 1 teaspoon finely chopped fresh rosemary

DIRECTIONS:

1. In a huge pot, heat the oil on high heat.
2. Reduce the heat to medium, and add the onion, garlic, salt, pepper, and red pepper flakes (if using). Sauté until the onion is golden, about 10 minutes.
3. Add the kale, and sauté until wilted, 1 to 2 minutes.
4. Pour the broth then bring to a boil.
5. Reduce the heat to simmer and cook until the kale is soft about 5 minutes.
6. Add the beans and rosemary. Cook until the beans are warmed through at least 2 to 3 minutes and serve.

Nutrition: Calories: 285 Fat: 15g Carbohydrates: 28g Sugar: 3g Fiber: 9g Protein: 13g Sodium: 1368mg

Meat & Poultry

81. Creamy Chicken

Preparation Time: 10 minutes
Cooking Time: 15 minutes
Servings: 2

INGREDIENTS:

- 3 tablespoon unsalted butter
- 2 pounds cut into 1-inch-thick strips skinless, boneless chicken breasts
- 4 minced garlic cloves
- ½ teaspoon ground ginger
- ½ teaspoon ground coriander
- ½ teaspoon ground cumin
- ¼ teaspoon crushed red pepper flakes
- ½ cup chicken broth
- 1/3 cup low-fat sour cream
- 1 tablespoon chopped fresh parsley

DIRECTIONS:

1. In a large skillet, melt butter on medium-high heat.
2. Add chicken and cook for about 5–6 minutes.
3. Add garlic and spices and cook for 1 minute.
4. Add broth and bring to a boil. Reduce the heat to medium-low.
5. Simmer for about 5 minutes, stirring occasionally.
6. Stir in cream and simmer, occasionally stirring for about 3 minutes.
7. Serve hot with the garnishing of parsley.

Nutrition: Calories: 206 Fat: 10.5g Carbs: 1.2g Protein: 26.1g Fiber: 0g Potassium: 43mg Sodium: 144mg

82. Grilled Chicken Pizza

Preparation Time: 20 minutes
Cooking Time: 15 minutes
Servings: 2

INGREDIENTS:

- 2 pita bread
- 3 tbsp. low sodium BBQ sauce
- 1/4 bowl red onion
- 4 oz. cooked chicken
- 2 tablespoon crumbled feta cheese
- 1/8 teaspoon garlic powder

DIRECTIONS:

1. Preheat oven at 350°F.
2. Place 2 pitas on the pan after you have put non-stick cooking spray on it.
3. Spread BBQ sauce (2 tablespoons) on the pita.
4. Cut the onion and put it on pita. Cube chicken and put it on the pitas.
5. Put also both feta and the garlic powder over the pita.
6. Bake for 12 minutes. Serve and enjoy!

Nutrition: Calories: 320 Protein: 22g Sodium: 520mg Potassium: 250mg Phosphorus: 220mg

83. Lemon & Herb Chicken Wraps

Preparation Time: 5 minutes
Cooking Time: 30 minutes
Servings: 2

INGREDIENTS:

- 4 oz. skinless and sliced chicken breasts
- 1/2 sliced red bell pepper
- 1 lemon
- 4 large iceberg lettuce leaves
- 1 tablespoon olive oil
- 2 tablespoons finely chopped fresh cilantro
- 1/4 teaspoon black pepper

DIRECTIONS:

1. Preheat the oven to 375°F.
2. Mix the oil, juice of ½ lemon, cilantro, and black pepper.
3. Marinate the chicken in the oil marinade, cover, and leave in the fridge for as long as possible.
4. Wrap the chicken in parchment paper, drizzling over the remaining marinade.
5. Place in the oven in an oven dish for 25-30 minutes or until chicken is thoroughly cooked through and white inside.
6. Divide the sliced bell pepper and layer it onto each lettuce leaf.
7. Divide the chicken onto each lettuce leaf and squeeze over the remaining lemon juice to taste.
8. Wrap and enjoy.

<u>Nutrition</u>: Calories: 364 Protein: 35g Carbohydrate: 32g Fat: 10g Sodium: 398mg Potassium: 413mg Phosphorus: 264mg

84. Cherry Chicken Salad

Preparation Time: 15 minutes
Cooking Time: 0 minutes
Servings: 2

INGREDIENTS:

- 2 cooked, boneless chicken breast halves, diced
- 1/3 cup dried cherries
- 1/3 cup diced celery
- 1/3 cup low-fat mayonnaise
- 1/3 cup cubed apples (optional)
- 1/2 teaspoon ground black pepper

DIRECTIONS:

1. In a large bowl, combine the dried cherries, chicken, celery, mayonnaise, and pepper and apple if desired.
2. Toss together well and refrigerate until chilled.
3. Serve

<u>Nutrition</u>: Calories: 281 Fat: 11.8g Cholesterol: 31mg Sodium: 586mg Dietary Fiber: 1.4g Sugars: 2.9g Protein: 14.7g Calcium: 12mg Potassium: 55mg Phosphorus: 20 mg

85. Southern Fried Chicken

Preparation Time: 5 minutes
Cooking Time: 26 minutes
Servings: 2

INGREDIENTS:

- 2 x 6-oz. boneless skinless chicken breasts
- 2 tablespoons hot sauce
- ½ teaspoon onion powder
- 1 tablespoon chili powder
- 2 oz. pork rinds, finely ground

DIRECTIONS:

1. Chop the chicken breasts in half lengthways and rub in the hot sauce. Combine the onion powder with the

chili powder, then rub it into the chicken. Leave to marinate for at least a half-hour.
2. Use the ground pork rinds to coat the chicken breasts in the ground pork rinds, covering them thoroughly. Place the chicken in your fryer.
3. Set the fryer at 350°F and cook the chicken for 13 minutes. Turn over the chicken and cook the other side for another 13 minutes or until golden.
4. Test the chicken with a meat thermometer. When fully cooked, it should reach 165°F. Serve hot, with the sides of your choice.

Nutrition: Calories: 408 Fat: 19 g Carbs: 10 g Protein: 35 g Phosphorus: 216 mg Potassium: 137 mg Sodium: 153 mg

86. Carrot & Ginger Chicken Noodles

Preparation Time: 5 minutes
Cooking Time: 10 minutes
Servings: 2

INGREDIENTS:

- 1 sliced green onion
- 2 teaspoon grated fresh ginger
- 4 oz. skinless sliced chicken breasts
- 1 lime
- 1 minced garlic clove
- 1 cup cooked rice noodles
- 1 teaspoon coconut oil
- 1 peeled and grated carrot

DIRECTIONS:

1. Heat a large pan over medium-high heat.
2. Add the coconut oil to a pan, and once melted, add the sliced chicken and brown for 4-5 minutes.
3. Now add the ginger and garlic and sauté for 4-5 minutes.
4. Add the green onion, carrot, and lime juice to the wok.
5. Put the cooked noodles in the pan and toss until hot through.
6. Serve hot and enjoy.

Nutrition: Calories: 187 Protein: 11 g Carbohydrate: 25 g Fat: 5 g Sodium: 39 mg Potassium: 91 mg Phosphorus: 178 mg

87. Cilantro Drumsticks

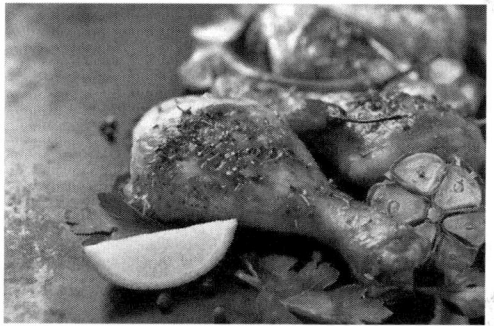

Preparation Time: 12 minutes
Cooking Time: 18 minutes
Servings: 2

INGREDIENTS:

- 8 chicken drumsticks
- ½ cup chimichurri sauce
- ¼ cup lemon juice

DIRECTIONS:

1. Coat the chicken drumsticks with chimichurri sauce and refrigerate in an airtight container for no less than an hour, ideally overnight.
2. When it's time to cook, pre-heat your fryer to 400°F.

3. Remove the chicken from the refrigerator and allow a return to room temperature for roughly twenty minutes.
4. Cook for eighteen minutes in the fryer. Drizzle with lemon juice to taste and enjoy.

Nutrition: Calories: 483 Fat: 29 g Carbs: 16 g Protein: 36 g Calcium 38mg, Phosphorous 146mg, Potassium 227mg Sodium: 121 mg

88. Chicken Sauté

Preparation Time: 10 minutes
Cooking Time: 25 minutes
Servings: 2

INGREDIENTS:

- 4 oz. chicken fillet
- 4 Red bell peppers, peeled
- 1 bell pepper, chopped
- 1 teaspoon olive oil
- 1 cup of water
- 1 teaspoon salt
- 1 chili pepper, chopped
- ½ teaspoon saffron

DIRECTIONS:

1. Pour water into the pan and bring it to a boil.
2. Meanwhile, chop the chicken fillet.
3. Add the chicken fillet in the boiling water and cook it for 10 minutes or until the chicken is tender.
4. After this, put the chopped bell pepper and chili pepper in the skillet.
5. Add olive oil and roast the vegetables for 3 minutes.
6. Add chopped red bell peppers and mix up well.
7. Cook the vegetables for 2 minutes more.
8. Then add salt and ¾ cup of water from the chicken.
9. Add chopped chicken fillet and mix up.
10. Cook the sauté for 10 minutes over medium heat.

Nutrition: Calories: 192 Fat: 7.2 g Fiber: 3.8 g Carbs: 14.4 g Protein: 19.2 g Calcium: 79mg Phosphorous: 216mg Potassium: 227mg Sodium: 101 mg

89. Rosemary Chicken

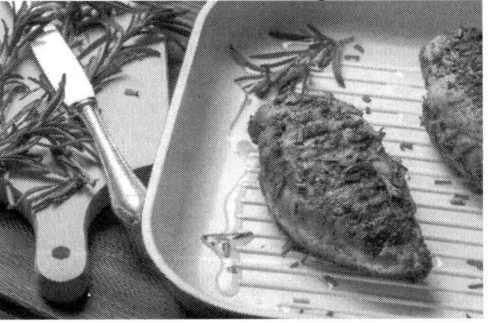

Preparation Time: 10 Minutes
Cooking Time: 10 Minutes
Servings: 2

INGREDIENTS:

- 2 zucchinis
- 1 carrot
- 1 teaspoon dried rosemary
- 4 chicken breasts
- 1/2 bell pepper
- 1/2 red onion
- 8 garlic cloves
- Olive oil
- 1/4 tablespoon ground pepper

DIRECTIONS:

1. Prepare the oven and preheat it at 375°F.
2. Slice both zucchini and carrots, add bell pepper, onion, garlic, and put all the ingredients, adding oil in a 13" x 9" pan.
3. Spread the pepper on the pan and roast for about 10 minutes.
4. Meanwhile, lift the chicken skin and spread black pepper and rosemary on the flesh.
5. Remove the vegetable pan from the oven and add the chicken, returning the pan to the range for about 30 more minutes. Serve and enjoy!

Nutrition: Calories: 215 Protein: 28 g Sodium: 105 mg Potassium: 580 mg Phosphorus: 250 mg

90. Chicken Strawberry Green Lettuce Salad with Ginger-Lime Dressing

Preparation Time: 10 minutes
Cooking Time: 30 minutes
Servings: 2

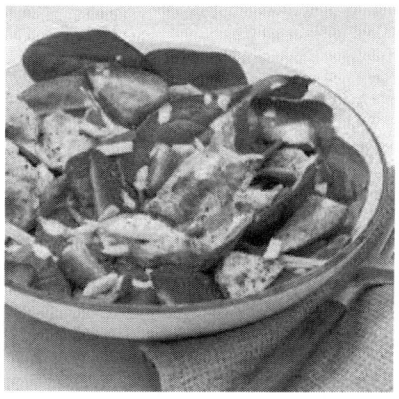

INGREDIENTS:

- 2 teaspoons. Corn oil
- 1 skinless, boneless chicken breast half-cut into bite-size pieces
- 1/2 teaspoon garlic powder
- 1 1/2 tablespoons. Mayonnaise
- 1/2 lime, juiced
- 1/2 teaspoon ground ginger
- 2 teaspoons. Almond milk
- 2cupfresh green lettuce stems removed
- 4 fresh strawberries, sliced
- 1 1/2 tablespoons. Slivered almonds
- Freshly ground black pepper to taste

DIRECTIONS:

1. In a skillet, heat oil over medium heat. Add the chicken breast and garlic powder. Cook the chicken for 10 minutes per side. When the juices run clear, remove from heat and set aside.
2. Combine the lime juice, almond milk, mayonnaise, and ginger in a bowl.
3. Place the green lettuce on serving dishes. Top with strawberries and chicken. Then sprinkle with almonds. Drizzle the salad with the dressing. Add pepper and serve.

Nutrition: Calories: 242 Fats: 17.3 g Carbohydrates: 7.5g Protein: 15.8 g Cholesterol: 40 mg Sodium: 117 mg Phosphorous 157mg Potassium 204mg

91. Creamy Turkey

Preparation Time: 12 minutes
Cooking Time: 10 minutes
Servings: 2
INGREDIENTS:

- 2 skinless, boneless turkey breast halves
- Salt and pepper to taste

- ½ teaspoon ground black pepper
- ½ teaspoon garlic powder
- 1 (10.75 ounces) can of chicken soup

DIRECTIONS:

1. Preheat oven to 375°F.
2. Clean turkey breasts and season with salt, pepper and garlic powder (or whichever seasonings you prefer) on both sides of turkey pieces.
3. Bake for 25 minutes, add chicken soup and bake for 10 more minutes (or until done). Serve over rice or egg noodles.

Nutrition: Calories: 160 Sodium: 157mg Dietary Fiber: 0.4g Sugars: 0.4g Protein: 25.6g Calcium: 2mg Potassium: 152mg Phosphorus: 85 mg

92. Parmesan And Basil Turkey Salad

Preparation Time: 15 minutes
Cooking Time: 35 minutes
Servings: 2

INGREDIENTS:

- 2 whole skinless, boneless turkey breasts
- salt and pepper to taste
- 1 cup mayonnaise
- 1 cup chopped fresh basil
- 2 cloves crushed garlic
- 3 stalks celery, chopped
- 2/3 cup grated Parmesan cheese

DIRECTIONS:

1. Season turkey with salt and pepper. Roast at 375°F for 35 minutes or until juices run clear. Let cool, and chop into chunks.
2. In a food processor, puree the mayonnaise, basil, garlic, and celery.
3. Combine the chunked turkey, pureed mixture, and Parmesan cheese; toss.
4. Refrigerate, and serve.

Nutrition: Calories: 303 Sodium: 190mg Dietary Fiber: 0.4g Sugars: 4.7g Protein: 8.5g Calcium: 73mg Potassium: 121mg Phosphorus: 100 mg

93. Oven-Baked Turkey Thighs

Preparation Time: 10 minutes
Cooking Time: 30 minutes
Servings: 2

INGREDIENTS:

- 10 ounces turkey thighs, skin on, bone-in
- 1/3 cup white wine
- 1 lemon
- 1 tablespoon fresh oregano
- 1/4 teaspoon cracked black pepper
- 1 tablespoon olive oil

DIRECTIONS:

1. Heat the oven to 350°F.
2. Add turkey thighs and white wine to an oven-proof pan. Squeeze half the lemon over turkey. Slice remaining lemon and top turkey with lemon slices.
3. Season turkey with fresh oregano, cracked pepper and olive oil.
4. Bake turkey for 25 to 30 minutes or until internal temperature reaches 165°F to 175°F.

Nutrition: Calories: 189 Sodium: 62mg Dietary Fiber: 0.9g Sugars: 0.6g Protein: 20.8g Calcium: 34mg Potassium: 232mg Phosphorus: 180 mg

94. Turkey Sausages

Preparation Time: 10 Minutes
Cooking Time: 10 Minutes
Servings: 2

INGREDIENTS:

- 1/4 teaspoon salt
- 1/8 teaspoon garlic powder
- 1/8 teaspoon onion powder
- 1 teaspoon fennel seed
- 1 pound 7% fat ground turkey

DIRECTIONS:

1. Press the fennel seed and in a small cup, put together turkey with fennel seed, garlic, onion powder, and salt.
2. Cover the bowl and refrigerate overnight.
3. Prepare the turkey with seasoning into different portions with a circle form and press them into patties ready to be cooked.
4. Cook at medium heat until browned.
5. Cook it for 1 to 2 minutes per side and serve them hot. Enjoy!

Nutrition: Calories: 55 Protein: 7 g Sodium: 70 mg Potassium: 105 mg Phosphorus: 75 mg

95. Pork with Bell Pepper

Preparation Time: 10 minutes
Cooking Time: 13 minutes
Servings: 2

INGREDIENTS:

- 1 tablespoon fresh ginger, chopped finely
- 4 garlic cloves, chopped finely
- 1 cup fresh cilantro, chopped and divided
- 1/4 cup olive oil, divided
- 1-pound tender pork, trimmed, sliced thinly
- 2 onions, thinly sliced
- 1 green bell pepper sliced thinly
- 1 tablespoon fresh lime juice

DIRECTIONS:

1. In a substantial bowl, mix ginger, garlic, 1/2 cup of cilantro, and 1/4 cup of oil.
2. Add pork and coat with mixture generously.
3. Refrigerate to marinate for approximately a couple of hours.
4. Heat a big skillet on medium-high heat.
5. Add pork mixture and stir-fry for approximately 4-5 minutes.
6. Transfer the pork right into a bowl.
7. In the same skillet, heat the remaining oil on medium heat.
8. Add onion and sauté for approximately 3 minutes.
9. Stir in bell pepper and stir-fry for about 3 minutes.
10. Stir in pork, lime juice, and remaining cilantro and cook for about 2 minutes. Serve hot.

Nutrition: Calories: 362 Fat: 13g Carbohydrates: 38g Fiber: 5g Protein: 21.8g Sodium: 399.1 mg Potassium: 421.7 mg Phosphorus: 169 mg

96. Pork Loins with Leeks

Preparation Time: 10 minutes
Cooking Time: 35 minutes
Servings: 2

INGREDIENTS:

- 1 sliced leek
- 1 tablespoon mustard seeds
- 6-ounce pork tenderloin
- 1 tablespoon cumin seeds
- 1 tablespoon dry mustard
- 1 tablespoon extra-virgin oil

DIRECTIONS:

1. Preheat the broiler to medium-high heat. In a dry skillet, heat mustard and cumin seeds until they start to pop (3-5 minutes). Grind seeds using a pestle and mortar or blender and then mix in the dry mustard.
2. Massage the pork on all sides using the mustard blend and add to a baking tray to broil for 25-30 minutes or until cooked through. Turn once halfway through.
3. Remove and place to one side, then heat-up the oil in a pan on medium heat and add the leeks for 5-6 minutes or until soft. Serve the pork tenderloin on a bed of leeks and enjoy it!

Nutrition: Calories: 139 Fat: 5g Carbohydrate: 2g Phosphorus: 278mg Potassium: 45mg Sodium: 47mg Protein: 18g

97. Chinese Beef Wraps

Preparation Time: 10 minutes
Cooking Time: 30 minutes
Servings: 2

INGREDIENTS:

- 2 iceberg lettuce leaves
- ½ diced cucumber
- 1 teaspoon canola oil
- 5-ounce lean ground beef
- 1 teaspoon ground ginger
- 1 tablespoon chili flakes
- 1 minced garlic clove
- 1 tablespoon rice wine vinegar

DIRECTIONS:

1. Mix the ground meat with the garlic, rice wine vinegar, chili flakes, and ginger in a bowl. Heat-up oil in a skillet over medium heat.
2. Put the beef in the pan and cook for 20-25 minutes or until cooked through. Serve beef mixture with diced cucumber in each lettuce wrap and fold.

Nutrition: Calories: 156 Fat: 2g Carbohydrate: 4 g Phosphorus: 1 mg Sodium: 54mg Protein: 14g Potassium: 0mg

98. Beef Ragu

Preparation Time: 10 minutes
Cooking Time: 10 minutes
Servings: 2

INGREDIENTS:

- 1/4 cup packaged pesto
- 1 teaspoon salt
- 2 large zucchinis, cut into noodle strips
- 1 tablespoon olive oil
- 1/4-pound ground beef
- 4 tablespoons fresh parsley, chopped

DIRECTIONS:

1. Heat the oil in a skillet under medium flame and cook the ground beef until thoroughly cooked, around 5 minutes. Discard excess fat.
2. Add the packaged pesto sauce and season with salt. Add t
3. Then chopped parsley and cook for three more minutes. Set aside.
4. In the same saucepan, place the zucchini noodles and cook for five minutes. Turn off the heat then add the cooked meat. Mix well.
5. Serve and enjoy.

Nutrition: Calories: 353 Fat: 30g Saturated Fat 6g Total Carbs: 2g Net Carbs: 1.3g Protein: 19g Sugar: 0.3g Fiber: 0.7g Sodium: 1481mg Potassium: 341mg

99. Country Fried Steak

Preparation Time: 10 minutes
Cooking Time: 1 hour and 40 minutes
Servings: 2

INGREDIENTS:

- 1 large onion
- 1/2 cup flour
- 3 tablespoons. vegetable oil
- 1/4 teaspoon pepper
- 11/2 pounds round steak
- 1/2 teaspoon paprika

DIRECTIONS:

1. Trim excess fat from steak
2. Cut into small pieces
3. Combine flour, paprika and pepper and mix together
4. Preheat skillet with oil
5. Cook steak on both sides
6. When the color of steak is brown remove to a platter
7. Add water (150 ml) and stir around the skillet
8. Return browned steak to skillet, if necessary, add water again so that bottom side of steak does not stick

Nutrition: Calories: 248 Protein: 30 g Fat: 10 g Carbohydrate: 5 g Phosphorus: 190 mg Potassium: 338 mg Sodium: 60 mg

100. Beef Pot Roast

Preparation Time: 20 minutes
Cooking Time: 1 hour
Servings: 2

INGREDIENTS:

- Round bone roast
- 2 - 4 pounds chuck roast

DIRECTIONS:

1. Trim off excess fat
2. Place a tablespoon of oil in a large skillet and heat to medium
3. Roll pot roast in flour and brown on all sides in a hot skillet
4. After the meat gets a brown color, reduce heat to low
5. Season with pepper and herbs and add 1/2 cup of water
6. Cook slowly for 11/2 hours or until it looks ready

Nutrition: Calories: 157 Protein: 24 g Fat: 13 g Carbs: 0 g Phosphorus: 204 mg Sodium: 50 mg

101. Homemade Burgers

Preparation Time: 10 minutes
Cooking Time: 20 minutes
Servings: 2

INGREDIENTS:

- 4 ounce lean 100% ground beef
- 1 teaspoon black pepper
- 1 garlic clove, minced
- 1 teaspoon olive oil
- 1/4 cup onion, finely diced
- 1 tablespoon balsamic vinegar
- 1/2 ounce brie cheese, crumbled
- 1 teaspoon mustard

DIRECTIONS:

1. Season ground beef with pepper and then mix in minced garlic.
2. Form burger shapes with the ground beef using the palms of your hands.
3. Heat a skillet on a medium to high heat, and then add the oil.
4. Sauté the onions for 5-10 minutes until browned.
5. Then add the balsamic vinegar and sauté for another 5 minutes.
6. Remove and set aside.
7. Add the burgers to the pan and heat on the same heat for 5-6 minutes before flipping and heating for a further 5-6 minutes until cooked through.
8. Spread the mustard onto each burger.
9. Crumble the brie cheese over each burger and serve!
10. Try with a crunchy side salad!
11. Tip: If using fresh beef and not defrosted, prepare double the ingredients and freeze burgers in plastic wrap (after cooling) for up to 1 month.
12. Thoroughly defrost before heating through completely in the oven to serve.

Nutrition: Calories: 178 Fat: 10g Carbohydrates: 4g Phosphorus: 147mg Potassium: 272mg Sodium: 273 mg Protein: 16g

102. Roast Beef

Preparation Time: 25 minutes
Cooking Time: 55 minutes
Servings: 2

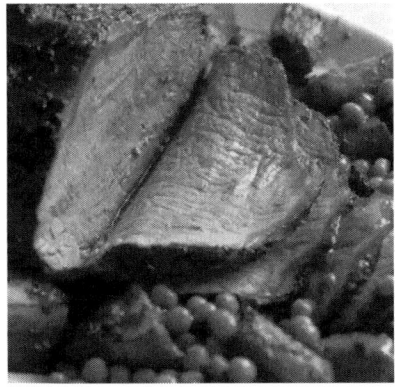

Preparation Time: 25 minutes
Cooking Time: 55 minutes
Servings: 2

INGREDIENTS:

- 3 pcs. quality rump or sirloin tip roast
- 1 cup pepper & herbs

DIRECTIONS:

1. Place in a roasting pan on a shallow rack. Season with pepper and herbs. Insert meat thermometer in the center or thickest part of the roast.

2. Roast to the desired degree of doneness. After removing over for about 15 minutes, let it chill. In the end, the roast should be moister than well done.

Nutrition: Calories: 158 Fat: 6 g Carbs: 0 g Protein: 24 g Phosphorus: 20 mg Potassium: 328 mg Sodium: 55 mg

103. Ginger & Bean Sprout Steak Stir-Fry

Preparation Time: 4 minutes
Cooking Time: 10 minutes
Servings: 2

INGREDIENTS:

- 2 teaspoons Grated fresh ginger
- 1 teaspoon coconut oil
- 1 teaspoon nutmeg
- 1 finely sliced green onion
- ¼ cup bean sprouts
- 5 oz. sliced lean organic beef steak
- 1 minced garlic clove

DIRECTIONS:

1. Add the strip beef into a dry, hot pan and cook for 4-5 minutes on each side or until they're cooked to your liking. Set aside.
2. Add the oil to a clean pan and sauté the bean sprouts and onions with the ginger, garlic, and nutmeg for 1 minute.
3. Serve the beef strips on a bed of vegetables and enjoy.

Nutrition: Calories: 227 Protein: 13 g Carbohydrate: 13 g Fat: 23 g Sodium: 50 mg Potassium: 258 mg Phosphorus: 170 mg

104. Beef Brochettes

Preparation Time: 20 minutes
Cooking Time: 20 minutes
Servings: 2

INGREDIENTS:

- 1 1/2 cups pineapple chunks
- 1 large sliced onion
- 2 lbs. thick steak
- 1 sliced medium bell pepper

For the marinade:

- 1 bay leaf
- 1/4 cup of vegetable oil
- 1/2 cup lemon juice
- 2 crushed garlic cloves

DIRECTIONS:

1. Cut beef cubes and place in a plastic bag
2. Combine marinade ingredients in a small bowl
3. Mix and pour over beef cubes
4. Seal the bag and keep in the refrigerator for 3 to 5 hours
5. Divide ingredients: onion, beef cube, green pepper, pineapple
6. Grill about 9 minutes each side

Nutrition: Calories: 304 Protein: 35 g Fat: 15 g Carbohydrate: 11 g Sodium: 70 mg Potassium: 388 mg Phosphorus 264 mg

105. Lamb with Prunes

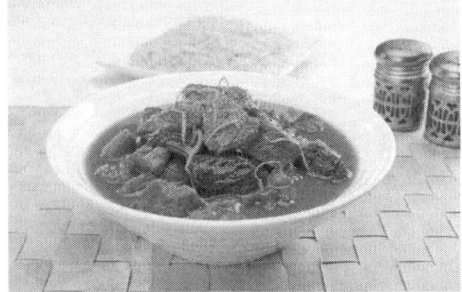

Preparation Time: 15 minutes
Cooking Time: 40 minutes
Servings: 2

INGREDIENTS:

- 3 tablespoons coconut oil
- 2 onions, chopped finely
- 1 (1-inch) piece fresh ginger, minced
- 3 garlic cloves, minced
- 1/2 teaspoon ground turmeric
- 2 1/2-pound lamb shoulder, trimmed and cubed into 3-inch size
- Salt to taste
- Ground black pepper to taste
- 1/2 teaspoon saffron threads, crumbled
- 1 cinnamon stick
- 3 cups of water
- 1 cup prunes, pitted and halved

DIRECTIONS:

1. In a big pan, melt coconut oil on medium heat.
2. Add onions, ginger, garlic cloves, and turmeric and sauté for about 3-5 minutes.
3. Put salt and black pepper in the lamb evenly.
4. In the pan, add lamb and saffron threads and cook for approximately 4-5 minutes.
5. Add cinnamon stick and water and produce to some boil on high heat.
6. Simmer until the lamb's desired doneness.
7. Stir in prunes and simmer.
8. Remove cinnamon stick and serve hot.

Nutrition: Calories: 225.6 Fat: 10g Carbohydrates: 8.5g Fiber: 1.7g Protein: 24g Sodium: 142mg Potassium: 439mg Phosphorus: 220mg

106. Spiced Lamb Burgers

Preparation Time: 10 minutes
Cooking Time: 20 minutes
Servings: 2

INGREDIENTS:

- 1 tablespoon extra-virgin olive oil
- 1 teaspoon cumin
- ½ finely diced red onion
- 1 minced garlic clove
- 1 teaspoon harissa spices
- 1 cup arugula
- 1 juiced lemon
- 6-ounce lean ground lamb
- 1 tablespoon parsley
- ½ cup low-fat plain yogurt

DIRECTIONS:

1. Preheat the broiler on medium to high heat. Mix the ground lamb, red onion, parsley, Harissa spices, and olive oil until combined.
2. Shape 1-inch-thick patties using wet hands. Add the patties to a baking tray and place under the broiler for 7-8 minutes on each side. Mix the yogurt, lemon juice, and cumin and serve over

the lamb burgers with arugula's side salad.

Nutrition: Calories: 306 Fat: 20g Carbohydrate: 10g Phosphorus: 269mg Potassium: 492mg Sodium: 86mg Protein: 23g

107. Lamb with Zucchini & Couscous

Preparation Time: 15 minutes
Cooking Time: 8 minutes
Servings: 2

INGREDIENTS:

- ¾ cup couscous
- ¾ cup boiling water
- 1/4 cup fresh cilantro, chopped
- 1 tablespoon olive oil
- 5-ounces lamb leg steak, cubed into ¾-inch size
- 1 medium zucchini, sliced thinly
- 1 medium red onion, cut into wedges
- 1 teaspoon ground cumin
- 1 teaspoon ground coriander
- 1/4 teaspoon red pepper flakes, crushed
- Salt, to taste
- 1/4 cup plain Greek yogurt
- 1 garlic herb, minced

DIRECTIONS:

1. In a bowl, add couscous and boiling water and stir to combine,
2. Cover whilst aside approximately 5 minutes.
3. Add cilantro and with a fork, fluff completely.
4. Meanwhile in a substantial skillet, heat oil on high heat.
5. Add lamb and stir fry for about 2-3 minutes.
6. Add zucchini and onion and stir fry for about 2 minutes.
7. Stir in spices and stir fry for about 1 minute
8. Add couscous and stir fry approximately 2 minutes.
9. In a bowl, mix together yogurt and garlic.
10. Divide lamb mixture in serving plates evenly.
11. Serve using the topping of yogurt.

Nutrition: Calories: 392 Fat: 5g Carbohydrates: 2g Fiber: 12g Protein: 35g

Seafood

108. Shrimp Paella

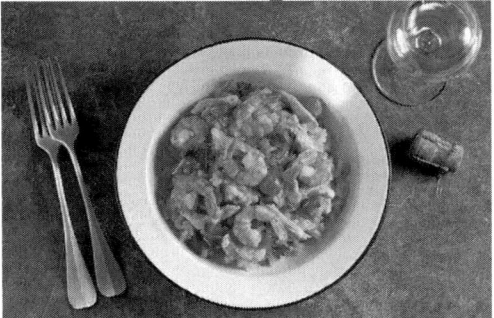

Preparation Time: 5 minutes
Cooking Time: 10 minutes
Servings: 2

INGREDIENTS:

- 1 cup cooked brown rice
- 1 chopped red onion
- 1 teaspoon paprika
- 1 chopped garlic clove
- 1 tablespoon olive oil
- 6 oz. frozen cooked shrimp
- 1 deseeded and sliced chili pepper
- 1 tablespoon oregano.

DIRECTIONS:

1. Heat the olive oil in a large pan on medium-high heat.
2. Add the onion and garlic and sauté for 2-3 minutes until soft.
3. Now add the shrimp and sauté for a further 5 minutes or until hot through.
4. Now add the herbs, spices, chili, and rice with 1/2 cup boiling water.
5. Stir until everything is warm, and the water has been absorbed.
6. Plate up and serve.

Nutrition: Calories: 221 Protein: 17g Sodium: 235mg Potassium: 176mg Phosphorus: 189mg.

109. Salmon & Pesto Salad

Preparation Time: 5 minutes
Cooking Time: 15 minutes
Servings: 2

INGREDIENTS:

For the Pesto:

- 1 minced garlic clove
- ½ cup fresh arugula
- ¼ cup extra virgin olive oil l
- ½ cup fresh basil
- 1 teaspoon black pepper

For the Salmon:

- 4 oz. skinless salmon fillet
- 1 tablespoon coconut oil.

For the Salad:

- ½ juiced lemon
- 2 sliced radishes
- ½ cup iceberg lettuce
- 1 teaspoon black pepper.

DIRECTIONS:

1. Prepare the pesto by blending all the pesto ingredients in a food processor or by grinding with a pestle and mortar. Set aside.
2. Add a skillet to the stove on medium-high heat and melt the coconut oil.
3. Add the salmon to the pan.
4. Cook for 7-8 minutes and turn over.

5. Cook for a further 3-4 minutes or until cooked through.
6. Remove fillets from the skillet and allow to rest.
7. Mix the lettuce and the radishes and squeeze over the juice of ½ lemon.
8. Flake the salmon with a fork and mix through the salad.
9. Toss to coat and sprinkle with a little black pepper to serve.

Nutrition: Calories: 221 Protein: 13g Carbs: 1g Fat: 34g Sodium: 80mg Potassium: 119mg Phosphorus: 158mg.

110. Baked Fennel & Garlic Sea Bass

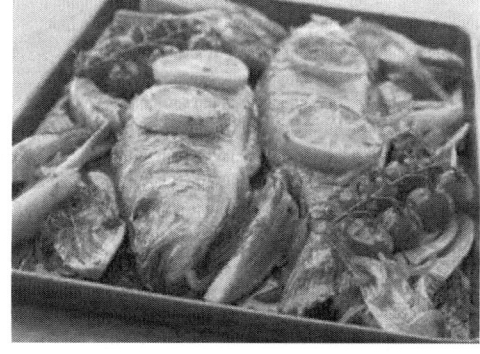

Preparation Time: 5 minutes
Cooking Time: 15 minutes
Servings: 2

INGREDIENTS:

- 1 lemon
- ½ sliced fennel bulb
- 6 oz. sea bass fillets
- 1 teaspoon black pepper
- 2 garlic cloves.

DIRECTIONS:

1. Preheat the oven to 375°F. Sprinkle black pepper over the Sea Bass. Slice the fennel bulb and garlic cloves. Add 1 salmon fillet and half the fennel and garlic to one sheet of baking paper or tin foil. Squeeze in 1/2 lemon juices. Repeat for the other fillet. Fold and add to the oven for 12-15 minutes or until fish is thoroughly cooked through.
2. Meanwhile, add boiling water to your couscous, cover, and allow to steam.
3. Serve with your choice of rice or salad.

Nutrition: Calories: 221 Protein: 14g Carbs: 3g Fat: 2g Sodium: 119mg Potassium: 398mg Phosphorus: 149mg.

111. 4-Ingredients Salmon Fillet

Preparation Time: 5 minutes
Cooking Time: 25 minutes
Servings: 2

INGREDIENTS:

- 4 oz. salmon fillet
- ½ teaspoon salt
- 1 teaspoon sesame oil
- ½ teaspoon sage.

DIRECTIONS:

1. Rub the fillet with salt and sage. Place the fish in the tray and sprinkle it with sesame oil. Cook the fish for 25 minutes at 365°F. Flip the fish carefully onto another side after 12 minutes of cooking.

Nutrition: Calories: 191 Fat: 11.6g Fiber: 0.1g Carbs: 0.2g Protein: 22g Potassium: 189 mg Sodium: 27 mg Phosphorus: 182 mg

112. Spanish Cod in Sauce

Preparation Time: 10 minutes
Cooking Time: 5.5 hours
Servings: 2

INGREDIENTS:

- 1 teaspoon tomato paste
- 1 teaspoon garlic, diced
- 1 white onion, sliced
- 1 jalapeno pepper, chopped
- 1/3 cup chicken stock
- 7 oz. Spanish cod fillet
- 1 teaspoon paprika
- 1 teaspoon salt.

DIRECTIONS:

1. Pour chicken stock into the saucepan.
2. Add tomato paste and mix up the liquid until homogenous.
3. Add garlic, onion, jalapeno pepper, paprika, and salt.
4. Bring the liquid to boil and then simmer it.
5. Chop the cod fillet and add it to the tomato liquid.
6. Close the lid and simmer the fish for 10 minutes over the low heat.
7. Serve the fish in the bowls with tomato sauce.

Nutrition: Calories: 113 Fat: 1.2g Fiber: 1.9g Carbs: 7.2g Protein: 18.9g Phosphorus: 65 mg Potassium: 303 mg Sodium: 169 mg

113. Haddock & Buttered Leeks

Preparation Time: 5 minutes
Cooking Time: 15 minutes
Servings: 2

INGREDIENTS:

- 1 tablespoon unsalted butter
- 1 sliced leek
- ¼ teaspoon black pepper
- 2 teaspoons Chopped parsley
- 6 oz. haddock fillets
- ½ juiced lemon.

DIRECTIONS:

1. Preheat the oven to 375°F.
2. Add the haddock fillets to baking or parchment paper and sprinkle with the black pepper.
3. Squeeze over the lemon juice and wrap into a parcel.
4. Bake the parcel on a baking tray for 10-15 minutes or until the fish is thoroughly cooked through.
5. Meanwhile, heat the butter over medium-low heat in a small pan.
6. Add the leeks and parsley and sauté for 5-7 minutes until soft.
7. Serve the haddock fillets on a bed of buttered leeks and enjoy!

Nutrition: Calories: 124 Protein: 15g Carbs: 0g Fat: 7g Sodium: 161mg Potassium: 251mg Phosphorus: 220mg.

114. Thai Spiced Halibut

Preparation Time: 5 minutes
Cooking Time: 20 minutes
Servings: 2

INGREDIENTS:

- 2 tablespoons. coconut oil
- 1 cup white rice
- ¼ teaspoon black pepper

- ½ diced red chili
- 1 tablespoon fresh basil
- 2 pressed garlic cloves
- 4 oz. halibut fillet
- 1 halved lime
- 2 sliced green onions
- 1 lime leaf.

DIRECTIONS:

1. Preheat oven to 400°F.
2. Add half of the ingredients into baking paper and fold into a parcel.
3. Repeat for your second parcel.
4. Add to the oven for 15-20 minutes or until fish is thoroughly cooked through.
5. Serve with cooked rice.

Nutrition: Calories: 311 Protein: 16g Carbs: 17g Fat: 15g Sodium: 31mg Potassium: 418mg Phosphorus: 257mg.

115. Monkfish Curry

Preparation Time: 5 minutes
Cooking Time: 20 minutes
Servings: 2

INGREDIENTS:

- 1 garlic clove
- 3 finely chopped green onions
- 1 teaspoon grated ginger
- 1 cup water
- 2 teaspoons chopped fresh basil
- 1 cup cooked rice noodles
- 1 tablespoon coconut oil
- ½ sliced red chili
- 4 oz. monkfish fillet
- ½ finely sliced stick lemon-grass
- 2 tablespoons chopped shallots.

DIRECTIONS:

1. Slice the monkfish into bite-size pieces.
2. Using a pestle and mortar or food processor, crush the basil, garlic, ginger, chili, and lemon-grass to form a paste.
3. Heat the oil in a large wok or pan over medium-high heat and add the shallots.
4. Now add the water to the pan and bring to the boil.
5. Add the monkfish, lower the heat and cover to simmer for 10 minutes or until cooked through. Enjoy with rice noodles and scatter with green onions to serve.

Nutrition: Calories: 249 Protein: 12g Carbs: 30g Fat: 10g Sodium: 32mg Potassium: 398mg Phosphorus: 190mg.

116. Tuna Noodle Casserole

Preparation Time: 10 minutes
Cooking Time: 35 minutes
Servings: 2

INGREDIENTS:

- 2 ounces of wide uncooked egg noodles
- 5 ounces of canned tuna in water
- ½ cup of sour cream
- ¼ cup of cottage cheese
- ½ cup of fresh sliced mushrooms
- ½ cup of frozen green peas
- 1 tablespoon of unsalted butter
- ¼ cup of unseasoned bread crumbs

DIRECTIONS:

1. Preheat oven to 350° F
2. Boil egg noodles based on the package instructions and drain. Also, drain and flake the tuna
3. Combine and mix the sour cream, cottage cheese, mushrooms, tuna, and peas in a medium bowl
4. Stir the drained noodle into the tuna mixture, and place in a small casserole dish that has been sprayed with a non-stick cooking spray
5. Melt butter, stir into the bread crumbs, then sprinkle over the mixture of noodles in step 4
6. Bake for about 20 to 25 minutes or until the bread crumbs start to brown
7. Divide into two and serve

Nutrition: Calories: 415 Protein: 22g Carbohydrates: 39g Fat: 19g Cholesterol: 88mg Sodium: 266mg Potassium: 400mg Phosphorus: 306mg Fiber: 3.2g

117. Citrus Tuna Ceviche

Preparation Time: 5 minutes
Cooking Time: 0 minutes
Servings: 2

INGREDIENTS:

- 1 (5 oz.) drained and rinsed Low-sodium water-packed tuna
- 1 tablespoon Cilantro
- ½, diced red onion
- 1 teaspoon Black pepper
- 1 Lemon
- 1 teaspoon red wine vinegar
- 1 chopped red bell pepper

DIRECTIONS:

1. Add tuna together with the rest of the ingredients into a serving bowl, mix well, and cover with plastic wrap.
2. Marinate as long as possible.
3. Serve with a salad or sandwich.

Nutrition: Calories: 127 Fat: 1g Carbs: 10g Protein: 21g Sodium: 278mg Potassium: 149mg Phosphorus: 116mg

118. Cilantro and Chili Infused Swordfish

Preparation Time: 30 minutes
Cooking Time: 15 minutes
Servings: 2

INGREDIENTS:

- 2 (30 oz.) Swordfish fillets
- 4 teaspoons Fresh cilantro
- 1, finely diced Onion
- 1 teaspoon Brown sugar
- 1 diced red chili
- 1 Lemon
- 1 tablespoon Extra virgin olive oil
- 1 clove, minced Garlic

DIRECTIONS:

1. Soak vegetables in warm water.
2. Meanwhile, add fish to an oven-proof baking dish.
3. Whisk onion, cilantro, chili, sugar, lemon juice, oil, and garlic in another bowl.
4. Spill marinade over the swordfish and turn the fish over to coat both sides.
5. Refrigerate for 30 minutes or more.
6. Preheat the broiler to medium heat.

7. Place oven dish under the broiler for 6 to 7 minutes on each side or until fish flakes easily with a fork. Serve hot.

Nutrition: Calories: 340 Fat: 16g Carb: 25g Protein: 23g Sodium: 258mg Potassium: 243mg Phosphorus: 284mg

119. Cooked Tilapia with Mango Salsa

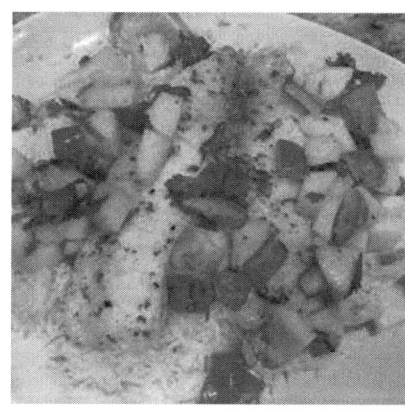

Preparation Time: 2 hours
Cooking Time: 10 minutes
Servings: 2

INGREDIENTS:

- 2 (3 oz. each) Fresh tilapia fillets
- ½, diced red onion
- ½, diced red bell pepper
- 2 tbsp. Fresh cilantro
- ¼ cup Olive oil
- 1 teaspoon Black pepper
- 1 Lime
- 4 Crackers/slices of melba toast

DIRECTIONS:

1. Preheat the broiler on medium heat.
2. Cut tilapia into small bite-size pieces.
3. Place tilapia under the broiler for 7 to 10 minutes or until cooked through.
4. Remove and allow to cool in a bowl. Then squeeze the juice from the lime over the top and mix well.
5. Mix the onion, bell pepper, cilantro, mango, pepper, and oil with the cooked tilapia and marinate for 2 hours in the refrigerator.
6. Divide into two bowls and serve with crackers.

Nutrition: Calories: 389 Fat: 29g Carbohydrate: 18g Protein: 17g Sodium: 134mg Potassium: 217mg Phosphorus: 183mg

120. Herb-Crusted Baked Haddock

Preparation Time: 10 minutes
Cooking Time: 20 minutes
Servings: 2

INGREDIENTS:

- ½ cup Breadcrumbs
- 3 tablespoons Chopped fresh parsley
- 1 tablespoon Lemon zest
- 1 teaspoon Chopped fresh thyme
- ¼ teaspoon Ground black pepper
- 1 tablespoon Melted unsalted butter
- 12-ounces, deboned and skinned Haddock fillets

DIRECTIONS:

1. Preheat the oven to 350°F.
2. In a bowl, stir together the parsley, breadcrumbs, lemon zest, thyme, and pepper until well combined.
3. Add the melted butter and toss until the mixture resembles coarse crumbs.

4. Place the haddock on a baking sheet and spoon the bread crumb mixture on top, pressing down firmly.
5. Bake the haddock in the oven for 20 minutes or until the fish is just cooked through and flakes off in chunks when pressed.

Nutrition: Calories: 143 Fat: 4g Carb: 10g Protein: 16g Sodium: 281mg Potassium: 285mg Phosphorus: 216mg

121. Baked Cod with Salsa

Preparation Time: 20 minutes
Cooking Time: 10 minutes
Servings: 2

INGREDIENTS:

For the salsa

- ½, chopped English cucumber
- 2 tablespoons Chopped fresh dill
- Juice of 1 lime
- Zest of 1 lime
- ¼ cup Boiled and minced red bell pepper
- ½ teaspoon Granulated sugar

For the fish

- 12 ounces, deboned and cut into 4 servings Cod fillets
- Juice of 1 lemon
- ½ teaspoon Ground black pepper
- 1 teaspoon Olive oil

DIRECTIONS:

1. To make the cucumber salsa: in a bowl, mix the salsa ingredients and set aside.
2. To make the fish: preheat the oven to 350°F.
3. Put the fish on a pie plate and add the lemon juice over the fillets.
4. Sprinkle with pepper and drizzle the olive oil evenly over the fillets.
5. Bake the fish for 6 minutes or until it flakes easily with a fork.
6. Transfer the fish to 4 plates and serve topped with cucumber salsa.

Nutrition: Calories: 110 Fat: 2g Carbohydrate: 3g Protein: 20g Sodium: 67mg Potassium: 275mg Phosphorus: 120mg

122. Cilantro-Lime Flounder

Preparation Time: 20 minutes
Cooking Time: 5 minutes
Servings: 2

INGREDIENTS:

- ¼ cup Homemade mayonnaise
- Juice of 1 lime
- Zest of 1 lime
- ½ cup Chopped fresh cilantro
- 4 (3-ounce) Flounder fillets
- Ground black pepper

DIRECTIONS:

1. Preheat the oven to 400°F.
2. In a bowl, stir together the cilantro, lime juice, lime zest, and mayonnaise.
3. Place 4 pieces of foil, about 8 by 8 inches square, on a clean work surface.
4. Place a flounder fillet in the center of each square.
5. Top the fillets evenly with the mayonnaise mixture.

6. Season the flounder with pepper.
7. Fold the foil's sides over the fish, create a snug packet, and place the foil packets on a baking sheet.
8. Bake the fish 5 minutes.
9. Unfold the packets and serve.

Nutrition: Calories: 92 Fat: 4g Carbohydrate: 2g Protein: 12g Sodium: 267mg Potassium: 137mg Phosphorus: 208mg

123. Halibut with Lemon Caper Sauce

Preparation Time: 10 minutes
Cooking Time: 10 minutes
Servings: 2

INGREDIENTS:

- 4 tablespoons lemon juice
- 1 tablespoon olive oil
- 20 oz. raw halibut steaks
- 2 tablespoons unsalted butter
- 2 teaspoons almond flour
- 1/2 cup reduced-sodium chicken broth
- 1/4 cup white wine
- 1 teaspoon capers
- 1/4 teaspoons white pepper

DIRECTIONS:

1. Season the halibut steaks with 2 tablespoons of lemon juice and olive oil in a bowl.
2. Now melt butter in the instant pot on Sauté mode.
3. Stir in the remaining ingredients and whisk well.
4. Place a steamer basket over the sauce mixture and add halibut to the basket.
5. Seal the lid and cook for 5 minutes on Manual mode at High pressure.
6. Once done, release the pressure completely, then remove the pot's lid.
7. Remove the fish and the basket.
8. Add the fish to the sauce and mix well gently. Serve warm.

Nutrition: Calories: 260 Fats: 10g Carbohydrate: 5g Protein: 36g Sodium: 118 mg Potassium: 573mg Phosphorus: 306mg

124. Jambalaya

Preparation Time: 10 minutes
Cooking Time: 25 minutes
Servings: 2

INGREDIENTS:

- 2 cups onion
- 1 cup bell pepper
- 2 garlic cloves
- 2 cups converted white rice, uncooked
- 1/2 teaspoons black pepper
- 8 oz. canned low-sodium tomato sauce
- 2 cups low-sodium beef broth
- 2 lbs. raw shrimp
- 1/2 cup margarine

DIRECTIONS:

1. Toss all the ingredients except margarine in a baking dish.
2. Place the margarine slice on top of the mixture.
3. Cover the dish with aluminum foil.
4. Pour 1.5 cups over into the instant pot and set the trivet over it.
5. Place the prepared baking dish over the trivet.

6. Press manual mode at high pressure and seal the lid. Cook for 25 minutes.
7. Once done, release the pressure and gently remove the pot's lid. Serve warm.

Nutrition: Calories: 207 Fats: 4g Carbohydrate: 30g Fiber: 1.5g Protein: 12g Sodium: 462mg Potassium: 304mg Phosphorus: 107mg

125. Shrimp Szechuan

Preparation Time: 10 minutes

Cooking Time: 9 minutes

Servings: 2

INGREDIENTS:

- 1 tablespoon canola oil
- 1/2 cup bean sprouts
- 1/2 cup green bell pepper, chopped
- 1/2 cup onion, chopped
- 1/2 cup raw mushroom pieces
- 1 teaspoon ginger root, grated
- 1/2 teaspoons garlic powder
- 1 tablespoon sesame oil
- 1 teaspoon red pepper flakes
- 1/3 cup low-sodium chicken broth
- 4 tablespoons sherry wine
- 1 teaspoon cornstarch
- 4 oz. shrimp, frozen

DIRECTIONS:

1. Start by heating oil in the Instant pot on Sauté mode.
2. Toss in onions, ginger, mushrooms, bell pepper, and bean sprouts.
3. Sauté for 2 minutes, then toss in all the ingredients except cornstarch.
4. Seal the lid and cook for 2 minutes on Manual mode at High pressure.
5. Release the pressure completely, then remove the pot's lid once done cooking.
6. Put and mix the cornstarch with 2 tablespoons water in a bowl.
7. Pour this mixture into the Instant pot and cook for 5 minutes on sauté mode. Serve warm.

Nutrition: Calories: 140 Fats: 4.3g Carbohydrate: 6g Fiber: 0.3g Protein: 19g Sodium: 372mg Potassium: 204.3 mg Phosphorus: 196mg

126. Baked Fish à la Mushrooms

Preparation Time: 10 minutes

Cooking Time: 17 minutes

Servings: 2

INGREDIENTS:

- 1 lb. fresh cod fillet
- 2 tablespoons margarine
- 1-1/2 cups sliced fresh mushrooms
- 1/4 cup white onion
- 1 teaspoon dried thyme

DIRECTIONS:

1. Arrange fish fillets in a baking dish suitable to fit the Instant Pot.
2. Melt margarine in a pan and add onion and mushroom.
3. Sauté this mixture for 5 minutes, then pour over the fish.
4. Drizzle crushed thyme on top of the sauce.
5. Pour 1 1/2 cups water and place a trivet over it.
6. Place the prepared baking dish over this trivet.

7. Cook for 12 minutes on Manual mode at High pressure.
8. Serve warm.

Nutrition: Calories: 155 Fats: 7 g Carbohydrate: 2 g Fiber: 0.5 g Protein: 21 g Sodium: 275 mg Potassium: 374 mg Phosphorus: 229 mg

127. Shrimp and Asparagus Linguine

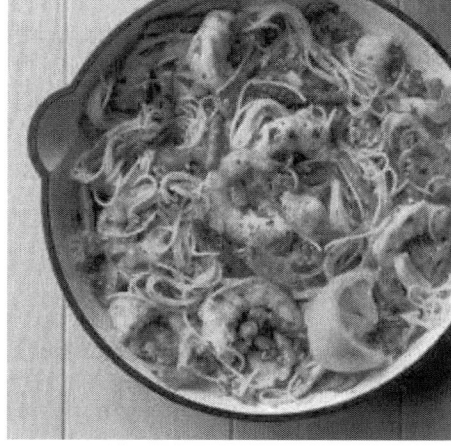

Preparation Time: 10 minutes
Cooking Time: 15 minutes
Servings: 2

INGREDIENTS:

- 8 oz. linguini, uncooked
- 1 tablespoon olive oil
- 1-3/4 cups asparagus
- 1/2 cup unsalted butter
- 2 garlic cloves
- 3 oz. cream cheese
- 3/4 teaspoons dried basil
- 2/3 cup dry white wine
- 1/2 lb. peeled, cooked shrimp

DIRECTIONS:

1. Prepare and cook the linguini as per the directions on the box and drain.
2. Put asparagus in a steamer basket and drizzle olive over it.
3. Pour 1.5 cup water into the Instant pot and set this basket inside.
4. Seal the lid and cook for 7 minutes on Manual mode at High pressure.
5. Release the pressure, then remove the pot's lid.
6. Slice the asparagus into small pieces.
7. Now melt butter in the Instant pot on sauté mode, after removing the water.
8. Stir in garlic and sauté for 1 minute, then add cream cheese.
9. Cook for 1 minute, then add basil.
10. Continue cooking for 5 minutes, then add white wine. Mix well and add asparagus and shrimp.
11. Toss and serve with cooked pasta.

Nutrition: Calories: 294 Fats: 9g Carbohydrate: 25g Fiber: 6g Protein: 30g Sodium: 389mg Potassium: 464.9mg Phosphorus: 362mg

128. Old Fashioned Salmon Soup

Preparation Time: 10 minutes
Cooking Time: 12 minutes
Servings: 2

INGREDIENTS:

- 2 tablespoons unsalted butter
- 1 medium carrot, diced
- 1/2 cup celery, chopped
- 1/2 cup onion, sliced
- 1 lb. sockeye salmon, cooked, diced
- 2 cups reduced-sodium chicken broth
- 2 cups almond milk
- 1/8 teaspoon black pepper
- 1/4 cup cornstarch

- 1/4 cup water

DIRECTIONS:

1. Start by melting the butter in the Instant Pot on Sauté mode.
2. Add all the veggies and sauté for 5 minutes.
3. Stir in all other ingredients except corn starch and water.
4. Seal the lid and cook for 2 minutes on Manual mode at High pressure.
5. Release the pressure, then remove the pot's lid once the cooking is done.
6. Mix cornstarch with the reserved water and pour it into the soup.
7. Stir cook for 5 minutes on sauté mode until it thickens. Serve warm.

Nutrition: Calories: 223 Fats: 1.7g Carbohydrate: 36g Fiber: 3.2g Protein: 14g Sodium: 822mg Potassium: 950mg Phosphorus: 82mg

129. Lemony Haddock

Preparation Time: 10 minutes
Cooking Time: 20 minutes
Serving: 2

INGREDIENTS:

- 1 tablespoon melted unsalted butter
- 12-ounces haddock fillets, deboned and skinned
- ½ cup breadcrumbs
- 3 tablespoons chopped fresh parsley
- 1 tablespoon lemon zest
- 1 teaspoon chopped fresh thyme
- ¼ teaspoon black pepper (ground)

DIRECTIONS:

1. Preheat the oven to 350°F.
2. In a mixing bowl, add breadcrumbs, parsley, lemon zest, thyme, and pepper. Combine to mix well.
3. Add butter and combine until you get crumbles.
4. Take a baking sheet and place haddock on it. Add crumb mixture on top.
5. Bake for 18-20 minutes until evenly brown from top.
6. Serve warm.

Nutrition: Calories: 183 Phosphorus: 233mg Potassium: 305mg Sodium: 316mg Protein: 16g

130. Glazed Salmon

Preparation Time: 10 minutes
Cooking Time: 10 minutes
Serving: 2

INGREDIENTS:

- 4 (3-ounce) salmon fillets
- 1 tablespoon olive oil
- 2 tablespoons honey
- 1 teaspoon lemon zest
- ½ teaspoon Black pepper (ground), to taste
- ½ scallion, chopped

DIRECTIONS:

1. Pat dry salmon with paper towels.
2. In a mixing bowl, add honey, lemon zest, and pepper. Combine to mix well.
3. Add salmon and coat evenly.
4. Take a medium saucepan or skillet, add oil. Heat over medium heat.

5. Add salmon and stir-cook until light brown and cooked well, for about 8-10 minutes. Flip in between.
6. Serve warm with scallions on top.

Nutrition: Calories: 238 Phosphorus: 220mg Potassium: 348mg Sodium: 74mg Protein: 16g

131. Tuna Casserole

Preparation Time: 15 minutes
Cooking Time: 35 minutes
Serving: 2

INGREDIENTS:

- ½ cup Cheddar cheese, shredded
- 2 tomatoes, chopped
- 7 oz tuna filet, chopped
- 1 teaspoon ground coriander
- ½ teaspoon salt
- 1 teaspoon olive oil
- ½ teaspoon dried oregano

DIRECTIONS:

1. Brush the casserole mold with olive oil.
2. Mix together chopped tuna fillet with dried oregano and ground coriander.
3. Place the fish in the mold and flatten well to get the layer.
4. Then add chopped tomatoes and shredded cheese.
5. Cover the casserole with foil and secure the edges.
6. Bake the meal for 35 minutes at 350°F.

Nutrition: 260 Calories - 56mg Phosphorus - 64mg Potassium - 29mg Sodium - 14.6mg Protein

132. Oregano Salmon with Crunchy Crust

Preparation Time: 10 minutes
Cooking Time: 2 hours
Serving: 2

INGREDIENTS:

- 8 oz salmon fillet
- 2 tablespoons panko breadcrumbs
- 1 oz Parmesan, grated
- 1 teaspoon dried oregano
- 1 teaspoon sunflower oil

DIRECTIONS:

1. In the mixing bowl combine panko breadcrumbs, Parmesan, and dried oregano.
2. Sprinkle the salmon with olive oil and coat in the breadcrumb's mixture.
3. After this, line the baking tray with baking paper.
4. Place the salmon in the tray and transfer to the oven preheated at 350°F.
5. Bake the salmon for 25 minutes.

Nutrition: Calories: 245 Phosphorus: 30mg Potassium: 67mg Sodium: 31mg Protein: 27.5g

133. Sardine Fish Cakes

Preparation Time: 10 minutes
Cooking Time: 10 minutes
Serving: 2

INGREDIENTS:

- 11 oz sardines, canned, drained
- 1/3 cup shallot, chopped
- 1 teaspoon chili flakes
- ½ teaspoon salt

- 2 tablespoon wheat flour, whole grain
- 1 egg, beaten
- 1 tablespoon chives, chopped
- 1 teaspoon olive oil
- 1 teaspoon butter

DIRECTIONS:

1. Heat up butter in the skillet.
2. Add shallot and cook it until translucent.
3. After this, transfer the shallot in the mixing bowl.
4. Add sardines, chili flakes, salt, flour, egg, chives, and mix up until smooth with the help of the fork.
5. Make the medium size cakes and place them in the skillet.
6. Add olive oil.
7. Roast the fish cakes for 3 minutes from each side over the medium heat.
8. Dry the cooked fish cakes with the paper towel if needed and transfer in the serving plates.

Nutrition: Calories: 221 Phosphorus: 36mg Potassium: 194mg Sodium: 31mg Protein: 21.3g

134. Cajun Catfish

Preparation Time: 10 minutes
Cooking Time: 10 minutes
Serving: 2

INGREDIENTS:

- 16 oz catfish steaks (4 oz each fish steak)
- 1 tablespoon Cajun spices
- 1 egg, beaten
- 1 tablespoon sunflower oil

DIRECTIONS:

1. Heat oil in a pan.
2. Meanwhile, dip every catfish steak in the beaten egg and coat in Cajun spices.
3. Place the fish steaks in the hot oil and roast them for 4 minutes from each side.
4. The cooked catfish steaks should have a light brown crust.

Nutrition: Calories: 263 Phosphorus: 39mg Potassium: 74mg Sodium: 20mg Protein:26g

135. Poached Gennaro/Seabass with Red Peppers

Preparation Time: 10 minutes
Cooking Time: 40 minutes
Serving: 2

INGREDIENTS:

- 2 red peppers, trimmed
- 11 oz Gennaro/seabass, trimmed
- 1 teaspoon salt
- ½ teaspoon ground black pepper
- 2 tablespoons butter
- 1 lemon

DIRECTIONS:

1. Remove the seeds from red peppers and cut them into wedges.
2. Then line the baking tray with parchment and arrange red peppers in a layer.
3. Rub Gennaro/seabass with ground black pepper and salt and place it on the peppers.
4. Then add butter.

5. Cut the lemon on the halves and squeeze the juice over the fish.
6. Bake the fish for 40 minutes at 350°F.

Nutrition: Calories: 148 Phosphorus: 36mg Potassium: 194mg Sodium: 31mg Protein: 8.5g

136. Oregano Grilled Calamari

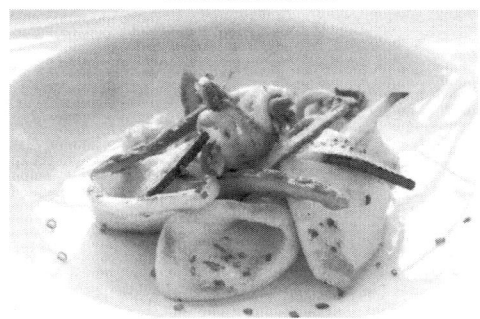

Preparation Time: 10 minutes
Cooking Time: 5 minutes
Serving: 2

INGREDIENTS:

- 2 teaspoons garlic, minced
- Pinch sea salt
- 2 tablespoons olive oil
- 2 tablespoons lemon juice
- 1 tablespoon chopped fresh parsley
- 1 tablespoon chopped fresh oregano
- Pinch black pepper (ground)
- ½ pound cleaned calamari
- Lemon wedges

DIRECTIONS:

1. Blend olive oil, lemon juice, parsley, oregano, garlic, salt, and pepper.
2. Add calamari and combine again. Refrigerate to marinate for 1 hour.
3. Preheat grill over medium heat setting; grease grates with some oil.
4. Grill calamari for 3 minutes, until evenly cooked. Turn halfway through.
5. Serve warm with some lemon wedges.

Nutrition: Calories: 103 Phosphorus: 103mg Potassium: 176mg Sodium: 73mg Protein: 4g

137. Nice Coconut Haddock

Preparation Time: 10 minutes
Cooking Time: 12 minutes
Servings: 2

INGREDIENTS:

- 4 haddock fillets, 5 ounces each, boneless
- 2 tablespoons coconut oil, melted
- 1 cup coconut, shredded and unsweetened
- ¼ cup hazelnuts, ground
- Salt to taste

DIRECTIONS:

1. Preheat your oven to 400 °F
2. Line a baking sheet with parchment paper
3. Keep it on the side
4. Pat fish fillets with a paper towel and season with salt
5. Take a bowl and stir in hazelnuts and shredded coconut
6. Drag fish fillets through the coconut mix until both sides are coated well
7. Transfer to a baking dish
8. Brush with coconut oil
9. Bake for about 12 minutes until flaky
10. Serve and enjoy!

Nutrition: Calories: 299 Fat: 24g Carbohydrates: 1g Protein: 20g Phosphorous 46mg, Potassium 86mg Sodium: 33 mg

Side Dishes

138. Cauliflower and Leeks

Preparation Time: 10 minutes

Cooking Time: 20 minutes

Servings: 2

INGREDIENTS:

- 1 and ½ cups leeks, chopped
- 1 and ½ cups cauliflower florets
- 2 garlic cloves, minced
- 1 and ½ cups artichoke hearts
- 2 tablespoons coconut oil, melted
- Black pepper to taste

DIRECTIONS:

1. Heat up a pan with the oil over medium-high heat, add garlic, leeks, cauliflower florets and artichoke hearts, stir and cook for 20 minutes.
2. Add black pepper, stir, divide between plates and serve.
3. Enjoy!

Nutrition: Calories: 192 Fat: 6,9 Fiber: 8,2 Carbohydrate: 35,1 Protein: 5,1 Phosphorus: 110mg Potassium: 117mg Sodium: 75mg

139. Eggplant and Mushroom Sauté

Preparation Time: 10 minutes

Cooking Time: 30 minutes

Servings: 2

INGREDIENTS:

- 2 pounds oyster mushrooms, chopped
- 6 ounces shallots, peeled, chopped
- 1 yellow onion, chopped
- 2 eggplants, cubed
- 3 celery stalks, chopped
- 1 tablespoon parsley, chopped
- A pinch of sea salt
- Black pepper to taste
- 1 tablespoon savory, dried
- 3 tablespoons coconut oil, melted

DIRECTIONS:

1. Heat up a pan with the oil over medium high heat, add onion, stir and cook for 4 minutes.
2. Add shallots, stir and cook for 4 more minutes.
3. Add eggplant pieces, mushrooms, celery, savory and black pepper to taste, stir and cook for 15 minutes.
4. Add parsley, stir again, cook for a couple more minutes, divide between plates and serve.
5. Enjoy!

Nutrition: Calories: 1013 Fat: 10,9 Fiber: 35,5 Carbohydrate: 156,5 Protein: 69,1 Phosphorus: 210mg Potassium: 217mg Sodium: 105mg

140. Mint Zucchini

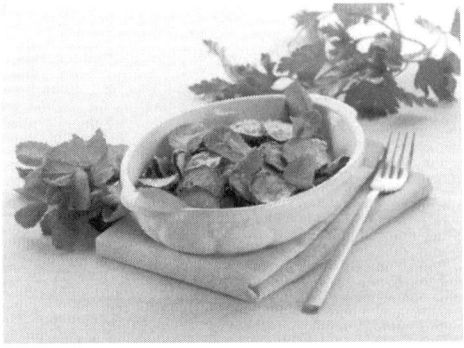

Preparation Time: 10 minutes

Cooking Time: 7 minutes
Servings: 2
INGREDIENTS:

- 2 tablespoons mint
- 2 zucchinis, halved lengthwise and then slice into half moons
- 1 tablespoon coconut oil, melted
- ½ tablespoon dill, chopped
- A pinch of cayenne pepper

DIRECTIONS:

1. Heat up a pan with the oil over medium-high heat, add zucchinis, stir and cook for 6 minutes.
2. Add cayenne, dill and mint, stir, cook for 1 minute more, divide between plates and serve.
3. Enjoy!

Nutrition: Calories: 46 Fat: 3,6 Fiber: 1,3 Carbohydrate: 3,5 Protein: 1,3 Phosphorus: 120mg Potassium: 127mg Sodium: 75mg

141. Celery and Kale Mix

Preparation Time: 10 minutes
Cooking Time: 20 minutes
Servings: 2
INGREDIENTS:

- 2 celery stalks, chopped
- 5 cups kale, torn
- 1 small red bell pepper, chopped
- 3 tablespoons water
- 1 tablespoon coconut oil, melted

DIRECTIONS:

1. Heat up a pan with the oil over medium-high heat, add celery, stir and cook for 10 minutes.
2. Add kale, water, and bell pepper, stir and cook for 10 minutes more.
3. Divide between plates and serve.
4. Enjoy!

Nutrition: Calories: 81 Fat: 3,5 Fiber: 1,8 Carbohydrate: 11,3 Protein: 2,9 Phosphorus: 120mg Potassium: 147mg Sodium: 75mg

142. Kale, Mushrooms and Red Chard Mix

Preparation Time: 10 minutes
Cooking Time: 17 minutes
Servings: 2
INGREDIENTS:

- ½ pound brown mushrooms, sliced
- 5 cups kale, roughly chopped
- 1 and ½ tablespoons coconut oil
- 3 cups red chard, chopped
- 2 tablespoons water
- Black pepper to taste

DIRECTIONS:

1. Heat up a pan with the oil over medium high heat, add mushrooms, stir and cook for 5 minutes.
2. Add red chard, kale and water, stir and cook for 10 minutes.
3. Add black pepper to taste, stir and cook 2 minutes more.
4. Divide between plates and serve.
5. Enjoy!

Nutrition: Calories: 97 Fat: 3,4 Fiber: 2,3 Carbohydrate: 13,3 Protein: 5,4 Phosphorus: 110mg Potassium: 117mg Sodium: 75mg

143. Bok Choy and Beets

Preparation Time: 10 minutes
Cooking Time: 30 minutes
Servings: 2

INGREDIENTS:

- 1 tablespoon coconut oil
- 4 cups bok choy, chopped
- 3 beets, cut into quarters and thinly sliced
- 2 tablespoons water
- A pinch of cayenne pepper

DIRECTIONS:

1. Put water in a large saucepan, add the beets, bring to a boil over medium heat, cover, and cook for 20 minutes and drain.
2. Heat up a pan with the oil over medium high heat, add the bok choy and the water, stir and cook for 10 minutes.
3. Add beets and cayenne pepper, stir, cook for 2 minutes more, divide between plates and serve as a side dish!
4. Enjoy!

Nutrition: Calories: 71 Fat: 3,7 Fiber: 2,2 Carbohydrate: 9 Protein: 2,3 Phosphorus: 110mg Potassium: 117mg Sodium: 75mg

144. Broccoli and Almonds Mix

Preparation Time: 10 minutes
Cooking Time: 11 minutes

Servings: 2

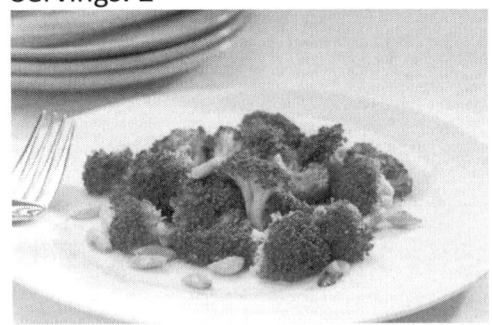

INGREDIENTS:

- 1 tablespoon olive oil
- 1 garlic clove, minced
- 1 pound broccoli florets
- 1/3 cup almonds, chopped
- Black pepper to taste

DIRECTIONS:

1. Heat up a pan with the oil over medium-high heat, add the almonds, stir, cook for 5 minutes and transfer to a bowl,
2. Heat up the same pan again over medium-high heat, add broccoli and garlic, stir, cover and cook for 6 minutes more.
3. Add the almonds and black pepper to taste, stir, divide between plates and serve.
4. Enjoy!

Nutrition: Calories: 116 Fat: 7,8 Fiber: 4 Carbohydrate: 9,5 Protein: 4,9 Phosphorus: 110mg Potassium: 117mg Sodium: 75mg

145. Squash and Cranberries

Preparation Time: 10 minutes
Cooking Time: 30 minutes
Servings: 2

INGREDIENTS:

- 1 tablespoon coconut oil
- 1 butternut squash, peeled and cubed
- 2 garlic cloves, minced
- 1 small yellow onion, chopped
- 12 ounces coconut milk
- 1 teaspoon curry powder
- 1 teaspoon cinnamon powder
- ½ cup cranberries

DIRECTIONS:

1. Spread squash pieces on a lined baking sheet, place in the oven at 425 degrees F, bake for 15 minutes and leave to one side.
2. Heat up a pan with the oil over medium high heat, add garlic and onion, stir and cook for 5 minutes.
3. Add roasted squash, stir and cook for 3 minutes.
4. Add coconut milk, cranberries, cinnamon and curry powder, stir and cook for 5 minutes more.
5. Divide between plates and serve as a side dish!
6. Enjoy!

Nutrition: Calories: 518 Fat: 47,6 Fiber: 7,3 Carbohydrate: 24,9 Protein: 5,3 Phosphorus: 110mg Potassium: 117mg Sodium: 75mg

146. Creamy Chard

Preparation Time: 10 minutes
Cooking Time: 10 minutes
Servings: 2
INGREDIENTS:

- Juice of ½ lemon
- 1 tablespoon coconut oil
- 12 ounces coconut milk
- 1 bunch chard
- A pinch of sea salt
- Black pepper to taste

DIRECTIONS:

1. Heat up a pan with the oil over medium-high heat, add chard, stir and cook for 5 minutes.
2. Add lemon juice, a pinch of salt, black pepper, and coconut milk, stir and cook for 5 minutes more.
3. Divide between plates and serve as a side.
4. Enjoy!

Nutrition: Calories: 453 Fat: 47,4 Fiber: 4 Carbohydrate: 10,1 Protein: 4,2 Phosphorus: 130mg Potassium: 1127mg Sodium: 85mg

147. Dill Carrots

Preparation Time: 10 minutes
Cooking Time: 30 minutes
Servings: 2
INGREDIENTS:

- 1 tablespoon coconut oil, melted
- 2 tablespoons dill, chopped
- 1 pound baby carrots
- 1 tablespoon coconut sugar
- A pinch of black pepper to taste

DIRECTIONS:

1. Put carrots in a large saucepan, add water to cover, bring to a boil over medium-high heat, cover and simmer for 30 minutes.

2. Drain the carrots, put them in a bowl, add melted oil, black pepper, dill, and the coconut sugar, stir very well, divide between plates and serve.
3. Enjoy!

Nutrition: Calories: 85 Fat: 3,6 Fiber: 3,5 Carbohydrate: 13,4 Protein: 1 Phosphorus: 140mg Potassium: 147mg Sodium: 65mg

148. Thai-Style Eggplant Dip

Preparation Time: 10 minutes
Cooking Time: 30 minutes
Servings: 2

INGREDIENTS:

- 1 pound Thai eggplant (or Japanese or Chinese eggplant)
- 2 tablespoons rice vinegar
- 2 teaspoons sugar
- 1 teaspoon low-sodium soy sauce
- 1 jalapeño pepper
- 2 garlic cloves
- ¼ cup chopped basil
- Cut vegetables for serving

DIRECTIONS:

1. Preheat the oven to 475°F
2. Pierce the eggplant in several places with a skewer or knife. Place on a rimmed baking sheet and cook until soft, about 30 minutes.
3. Let cool, cut in half, and scoop out the flesh of the eggplant into a blender.
4. Add the rice vinegar, sugar, soy sauce, jalapeño, garlic, and basil to the blender. Process until smooth. Serve with cut vegetables

5. Lower sodium tip: If you need to lower your sodium further, omit the soy sauce to lower the sodium to 3mg.

Nutrition: Calories: 40 Total Fat: 0g Saturated Fat: 0g Cholesterol: 0mg Carbohydrates: 10g Fiber: 4g Protein: 2g Phosphorus: 34mg Potassium: 284mg Sodium: 47mg

149. Collard Salad Rolls with Peanut Dipping Sauce

Preparation Time: 10 minutes
Cooking Time: 10 minutes
Servings: 2

INGREDIENTS:

For the dipping sauce:

- ¼ cup peanut butter
- 2 tablespoons honey
- Juice of 1 lime
- ¼ teaspoon red chili flakes

For the salad rolls:

- 4 ounces' extra-firm tofu
- 1 bunch collard greens
- 1 cup thinly sliced purple cabbage
- 1 cup bean sprouts
- 2 carrots, cut into matchsticks
- ½ cup cilantro leaves and stems

DIRECTIONS:

To Make the Dipping Sauce:

1. In a blender, combine the peanut butter, honey, lime juice, chili flakes, and process until smooth. Put 1 to 2 tablespoons of water as desired for consistency.

To Make the Salad Rolls:

2. Using paper towels, press the excess moisture from the tofu. Cut into ½-inch-thick matchsticks.
3. Remove any tough stems from the collard greens and set aside.
4. Arrange all of the ingredients within reach. Cup one collard green leaf in your hand, and add a couple pieces of the tofu and a small amount each of the cabbage, bean sprouts, and carrots. Top with a couple cilantro sprigs and roll into a cylinder. Place each roll, seam-side down, on a serving platter while you assemble the rest of the rolls. Serve with the dipping sauce.
5. Substitution tip: To lower the potassium, limit the cabbage and use only 1 carrot, which will drop the potassium to 208mg.

Nutrition: Calories: 174 Total Fat: 9g Saturated Fat: 2g Cholesterol: 0mg Carbohydrates: 20g Fiber: 5g Protein: 8g Phosphorus: 56mg Potassium: 284mg Sodium: 42mg

150. Simple Roasted Broccoli

Preparation Time: 5 minutes
Cooking Time: 20 minutes
Servings: 2

INGREDIENTS:

- 2 small heads broccoli, cut into florets
- 1 tablespoon extra-virgin olive oil
- 3 garlic cloves, minced

DIRECTIONS:

1. Preheat the oven to 425°F.
2. Toss the broccoli with the olive oil and garlic.
3. Arrange in a single layer on a baking sheet.
4. Roast for 10 minutes, then flip the broccoli and roast an additional 10 minutes. Serve.
5. Cooking tip: Roasted broccoli makes for great leftovers—throw them in a quick salad for added flavor and bulk. To save leftovers, refrigerate in an airtight container for three to five days.

Nutrition: Calories: 38 Total Fat: 2g Saturated Fat: 0g Cholesterol: 0mg Carbohydrates: 4g Fiber: 1g Protein: 1g Phosphorus: 32mg Potassium: 150mg Sodium: 15mg

151. Roasted Mint Carrots

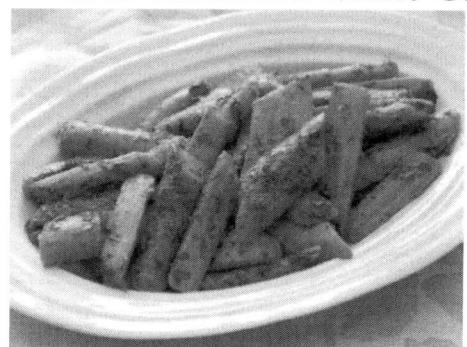

Preparation Time: 20 minutes
Cooking Time: 5 minutes
Servings: 2

INGREDIENTS:

- 1-pound carrots, trimmed
- 1 tablespoon extra-virgin olive oil
- Freshly ground black pepper
- ¼ cup thinly sliced mint

DIRECTIONS:

1. Preheat the oven to 425°F.
2. Assemble the carrots in a single layer on a rimmed baking sheet. Drizzle with the olive oil and shake the carrots on the sheet to coat. Season with pepper.
3. Cook for 20 minutes, or until tender and browned, stirring twice while cooking. Sprinkle with the mint and serve.
1. Substitution tip: To lower the potassium in this dish, use 8 ounces of carrots and 8 ounces of turnips cut into cubes. This will cut the potassium to 193mg.

Nutrition: Calories: 51 Total Fat: 2g Saturated Fat: 0g Cholesterol: 0mg Carbohydrates: 7g Fiber: 2g Protein: 1g Phosphorus: 26mg Potassium: 242mg Sodium: 52mg

152. Roasted Root Vegetables

Preparation Time: 10 minutes
Cooking Time: 25 minutes
Servings: 2

INGREDIENTS:

- 1 cup chopped turnips
- 1 cup chopped rutabaga
- 1 cup chopped parsnips
- 1 tablespoon extra-virgin olive oil
- 1 teaspoon fresh chopped rosemary
- Freshly ground black pepper

DIRECTIONS:

1. Preheat the oven to 420°F.
2. Toss the turnips, rutabaga, and parsnips with the olive oil and rosemary.
3. Assemble in a single layer on a baking sheet, and season with pepper.
4. Roast until the vegetables are tender and browned, 20 to 25 minutes, stirring once.

Nutrition: Calories: 52 Total Fat: 2g Saturated Fat: 0g Cholesterol: 0mg Carbohydrates: 7g Fiber: 2g Protein: 1g Phosphorus: 35mg Potassium: 205mg Sodium: 22mg

153. Vegetable Couscous

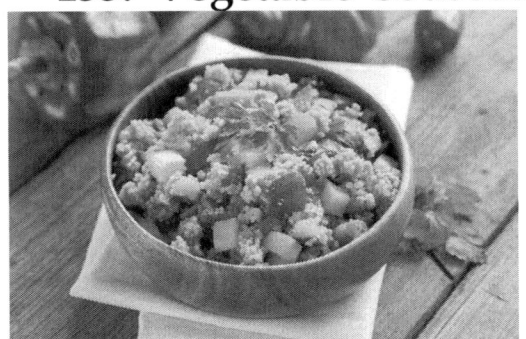

Preparation Time: 10 minutes
Cooking Time: 51 minutes
Servings: 2

INGREDIENTS:

- 1 tablespoon extra-virgin olive oil
- ½ sweet onion, diced
- 1 carrot, diced
- 1 celery stalk, diced
- ½ cup diced red or yellow bell pepper
- 1 small zucchini, diced
- 1 cup couscous
- 1½ cups Simple Chicken Broth or low-sodium store-bought chicken stock
- ½ teaspoon garlic powder
- Freshly ground black pepper

DIRECTIONS:

1. Place the onion, carrot, celery, bell pepper, and cook, stirring occasionally, until the vegetables are just becoming tender, about 5 to 7 minutes.
2. Add the zucchini, couscous, broth, and garlic powder.
3. Stir to blend and bring to a boil.
4. Cover and remove from the heat. Let stand for 5 to 8 minutes. Fluff with a fork, season with pepper, and serve.

Nutrition: Calories: 154 Total Fat: 3g Saturated Fat: 1g Cholesterol: 0mg Carbohydrates: 27g Fiber: 2g Protein: 5g Phosphorus: 83mg Potassium: 197mg Sodium: 36mg

154. Ginger Cauliflower Rice

Preparation Time: 10 minutes
Cooking Time: 10 minutes
Servings: 2

INGREDIENTS:

- 5 cups cauliflower florets
- 3 tablespoons coconut oil
- 4 ginger slices, grated
- 1 tablespoon coconut vinegar
- 3 garlic cloves, minced
- 1 tablespoon chives, minced
- A pinch of sea salt
- Black pepper to taste

DIRECTIONS:

1. Put cauliflower florets in a food processor and pulse well.
2. Heat up a pan with the oil over medium-high heat, add ginger, stir and cook for 3 minutes.
3. Add cauliflower rice and garlic, stir and cook for 7 minutes.
4. Add salt, black pepper, vinegar, and chives, stir, cook for a few seconds more, divide between plates and serve.
5. Enjoy!

Nutrition: Calories: 125 Fat: 10,4 Fiber: 3,2 Carbohydrate: 7,9 Protein: 2,7 Phosphorus: 110mg Potassium: 117mg Sodium: 75mg

155. Basil Zucchini Spaghetti

Preparation Time: 1 hour and 10 minutes
Cooking Time: 10 minutes
Servings: 2

INGREDIENTS:

- 1/3 cup coconut oil, melted
- 4 zucchinis, cut with a spiralizer
- ¼ cup basil, chopped
- A pinch of sea salt
- Black pepper to taste
- ½ cup walnuts, chopped
- 2 garlic cloves, minced

DIRECTIONS:

1. In a bowl, mix zucchini spaghetti with salt and pepper, toss to coat, leave aside for 1 hour, drain well and put in a bowl.
2. Heat up a pan with the oil over medium-high heat, add zucchini spaghetti and garlic, stir and cook for 5 minutes.

3. Add basil and walnuts and black pepper, stir and cook for 3 minutes more.
4. Divide between plates and serve as a side dish
5. Enjoy!

Nutrition: Calories: 287 Fat: 27,8 Fiber: 3,3 Carbohydrate: 8,7 Protein: 6,3 Phosphorus: 110mg Potassium: 117mg Sodium: 75mg

156. Braised Cabbage

Preparation Time: 10 minutes
Cooking Time: 10 minutes
Servings: 2

INGREDIENTS:

- 1 small cabbage head, shredded
- 2 tablespoons water
- A drizzle of olive oil
- 6 ounces shallots, cooked and chopped
- A pinch of black pepper
- A pinch of sweet paprika
- 1 tablespoon dill, chopped

DIRECTIONS:

1. Heat up a pan with the oil over medium heat, add the cabbage and the water, stir and sauté for 5 minutes.
2. Add the rest of the ingredients, toss, cook for 5 minutes more, divide everything between plates and serve as a side dish!
3. Enjoy!

Nutrition: Calories: 91 Fat: 0,5 Fiber: 5,8 Carbohydrate: 20,8 Protein: 4,1 Phosphorus: 120mg Potassium: 127mg Sodium: 75mg

Vegetarian & Vegan

157. Mixed Pepper Paella

Preparation Time: 10 minutes
Cooking Time: 35-40 minutes
Servings: 2

INGREDIENTS:

- 1 tablespoon extra-virgin olive oil
- ½ chopped red onion
- 1 lemon
- ½ chopped yellow bell pepper
- 1 cup homemade chicken broth
- ½ chopped zucchini
- 1 teaspoon dried oregano
- ½ chopped red bell pepper
- 1 teaspoon dried parsley
- 1 cup brown rice
- 1 teaspoon paprika

DIRECTIONS:

1. Add the rice to a pot of cold water and cook for 15 minutes.
2. Drain the water, cover the pan and leave to one side.
3. Heat the oil in a skillet over medium-high heat.
4. Add the bell peppers, onion and zucchini, sautéing for 5 minutes.
5. To the pan, add the rice, herbs, spices and juice of the lemon along with the chicken broth.
6. Cover and turn the heat right down and allow to simmer for 15-20 minutes.
7. Serve hot.

Nutrition: Calories: 210 Protein: 4 g Carbohydrate: 33 g Fat: 7 g Sodium: 20 mg Potassium: 33 mg Phosphorus: 156 mg

158. Minted Zucchini Noodles

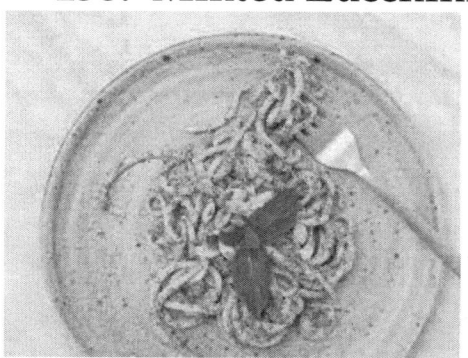

Preparation Time: 5 minutes
Cooking Time: 10 minutes
Servings: 2

INGREDIENTS:

- ¼ deseeded and chopped red chili
- 2 tablespoons Extra virgin olive oil
- ½ juiced lemon
- 4 peeled and sliced zucchinis
- ½ cup chopped fresh mint
- 1 tsp. black pepper
- ½ cup arugula

DIRECTIONS:

1. Whisk the mint, pepper, chili and olive oil to make a dressing.
2. Meanwhile, heat a pan of water on a high heat and bring to the boil.
3. Add the zucchini noodles and turn the heat down to simmer for 3-4 minutes.
4. Remove from the heat and place in a bowl of cold water immediately.
5. Toss the noodles in the dressing.

6. Mix the arugula with the lemon juice to serve on the top.
7. Enjoy!

Nutrition: Calories: 148 Protein: 2 Carbohydrate: 4 g Fat: 13 g Sodium: 7 mg Potassium: 422 mg Phosphorus: 256 mg

159. Vegan Alfredo Fettuccine Pasta

Preparation Time: 15 minutes
Cooking Time: 15 minutes
Servings: 2

INGREDIENTS:

- 2 medium white potatoes
- ¼ white onion
- 1 tablespoon Italian seasoning
- 1 teaspoon lemon juice
- 2 cloves garlic
- 1 teaspoon salt
- 12 ounces Fettuccine pasta
- ½ cup raw cashew

DIRECTIONS:

1. Start by placing a pot on high flame and boiling 4 cups of water.
2. Peel the potatoes and cut them into small cubes. Cut the onion into cubes as well.
3. Add the potatoes and onions to the boiling water and cook for about 10 minutes.
4. Remove the onions and potatoes. Keep aside. Save the water.
5. Take another pot and fill it with water. Season generously with salt.
6. Toss in the fettuccine pasta and cook as per package instructions.
7. Take a blender and add in the raw cashews, veggies, nutritional yeast, truffle oil, lemon juice and 1 cup of saved water. Blend into a smooth puree.
8. Add in the garlic and salt.
9. Drain the cooked pasta using a colander. Transfer into a mixing bowl.
10. Pour the prepared sauce on top of the cooked fettuccine pasta. Serve.
11. Nutritional yeast (optional) - 1 teaspoon
12. Truffle oil (optional) - ¼ teaspoon

Nutrition: Calories: 844 calories Fat: 13 g Carbohydrates: 152 g Protein: 28 g Phosphorus: 514 mg Potassium: 264 mg Sodium: 196 mg

160. Chinese Tempeh Stir Fry

Preparation Time: 5 minutes
Cooking Time: 15 minutes
Servings: 2 servings

INGREDIENTS:

- 2 oz. sliced tempeh
- 1 cup cooked rice
- 1 minced garlic clove
- ½ cup green onions
- 1 teaspoon minced fresh ginger
- 1 tablespoon coconut oil
- ½ cup corn

DIRECTIONS:

1. Heat the oil in a skillet or wok on high heat and add garlic and ginger.
2. Sauté for 1 minute.
3. Now add the tempeh and cook for 5-6 minutes before adding the corn for a further 10 minutes.

4. Now add the green onions and serve over rice.

Nutrition: Calories: 304 kcal Total Fat: 4 g Saturated Fat: 0 g Cholesterol: 0 mg Sodium: 91 mg Carbohydrate: 35 g Fiber: 0 g Sugar: 0 g Protein: 10 g Phosphorous: 234mg, Potassium: 169mg

161. Pesto Pasta Salad

Preparation Time: 15 minutes
Cooking Time: 15 minutes
Servings: 4

INGREDIENTS:

- 1 cup fresh basil leaves
- ½ cup packed fresh flat-leaf parsley leaves
- ½ cup arugula, chopped
- 2 tablespoons Parmesan cheese, grated
- ¼ cup extra-virgin olive oil
- 3 tablespoons mayonnaise
- 2 tablespoons water
- 12 ounces whole-wheat rotini pasta
- 1 red bell pepper, chopped
- 1 medium yellow summer squash, sliced
- 1 cup frozen baby peas

DIRECTIONS:

1. Boil water in a large pot.
2. Meanwhile, combine the basil, parsley, arugula, cheese, and olive oil in a blender or food processor. Process until the herbs are finely chopped. Add the mayonnaise and water, then process again. Set aside.
3. Prepare the pasta to the pot of boiling water; cook according to package directions, about 8 to 9 minutes. Drain well, reserving ¼ cup of the cooking liquid.
4. Combine the pesto, pasta, bell pepper, squash, and peas in a large bowl and toss gently, adding enough reserved pasta cooking liquid to make a sauce on the salad. Serve immediately or cover and chill, then serve.
5. Store covered in the refrigerator for up to 3 days.

Nutrition: Calories: 378 Fat: 24g Carbohydrates: 35g Protein: 9g Sodium: 163mg Potassium: 472mg Phosphorus: 213mg

162. Asparagus Fried Rice

Preparation Time: 10 minutes
Cooking Time: 10 minutes
Servings: 2

INGREDIENTS:

- 3 large eggs, beaten
- ½ teaspoon ground ginger
- 2 teaspoons low-sodium soy sauce
- 2 tablespoons olive oil
- 1 onion, diced
- 4 garlic cloves, minced
- 1 cup sliced cremini mushrooms
- 1 (10-ounce) package frozen white rice, thawed
- 8 ounces fresh asparagus, about 15 spears, cut into 1-inch pieces
- 1 teaspoon sesame oil

DIRECTIONS:

1. Whisk the eggs, ginger, and soy sauce in a small bowl and set aside.

2. Heat the olive oil in a medium skillet or wok over medium heat.
3. Add the onion and garlic and sauté for 2 minutes until tender-crisp.
4. Add the mushrooms and rice; stir-fry for 3 minutes longer.
5. Put asparagus and cook for 2 minutes.6.
6. Pour in the egg mixture. Stir the eggs until cooked through, 2 to 3 minutes, and stir into the rice mixture.
7. Sprinkle the fried rice with the sesame oil and serve.

Nutrition: Calories: 247 Fat: 13g Carbohydrates: 25g Protein: 9g Sodium: 149mg Potassium: 367mg Phosphorus: 206mg

163. Vegetarian Taco Salad

Preparation Time: 15 minutes
Cooking Time: 15 minutes
Servings: 2

INGREDIENTS:

- 1½ cups canned low-sodium or no-salt-added pinto beans, rinsed and drained
- 1 (10-ounce) package frozen white rice, thawed
- 1 red bell pepper, chopped
- 3 scallions, white and green parts, chopped
- 1 jalapeño pepper, minced
- 1 cup frozen corn, thawed and drained
- 1 tablespoon chili powder
- 1 cup chopped romaine lettuce
- 2 cups chopped butter lettuce
- ½ cup Powerhouse Salsa
- ½ cup grated pepper Jack cheese

DIRECTIONS:

1. Combine the beans, rice, bell pepper, scallions, jalapeño, and corn in a medium bowl.
2. Sprinkle with the chili powder and stir gently.
3. Stir in the romaine and butter lettuce.
4. Serve topped with Powerhouse Salsa and cheese.

Nutrition: Calories: 254 Fat: 7g Carbohydrates: 39g Protein: 11g Sodium: 440mg Potassium: 599mg Phosphorus: 240mg

164. Sautéed Green Beans

Preparation Time: 10 minutes
Cooking Time: 15 minutes
Servings: 2

INGREDIENTS:

- 2 cup frozen green beans
- ½ cup red bell pepper
- 4 teaspoons margarine
- ¼ cup onion
- 1 teaspoon dried dill weed
- 1 teaspoon dried parsley
- ¼ teaspoon black pepper

DIRECTIONS:

1. Cook green beans in a large pan of boiling water until tender, then drain.
2. While the beans are cooking, melt the margarine in a skillet and fry the other vegetables.
3. Add the beans to sautéed vegetables.
4. Sprinkle with freshly ground pepper and serve with meat and fish dishes.

Nutrition: Calories: 67 Carbohydrate: 8g Protein: 4g Sodium: 5mg Potassium: 179mg Phosphorous: 32mg

165. Garlicky Penne Pasta with Asparagus

Preparation Time: 10 minutes
Cooking Time: 10 minutes
Servings: 2

INGREDIENTS:

- 2 tablespoons butter
- 1lb asparagus, cut into 2-inch pieces
- 2 teaspoons lemon juice
- 4 cup whole wheat penne pasta, cooked
- ¼ cup shredded Parmesan cheese
- ¼ teaspoon Tabasco® hot sauce

DIRECTIONS:

1. Add olive oil and butter in a skillet over medium heat.
2. Fry garlic and red pepper flakes for 2-3 minutes.
3. Add asparagus, Tabasco sauce, lemon juice, and black pepper to skillet and cook for a further 6 minutes.
4. Add hot pasta and cheese. Toss and serve.

Nutrition: Calories: 387 Carbohydrate: 49g Protein: 13g Sodium: 93 Potassium: 258mg Phosphorous: 252mg

166. Garlic Mashed Carrots

Preparation Time: 5 minutes
Cooking Time: 20 minutes
Servings: 2

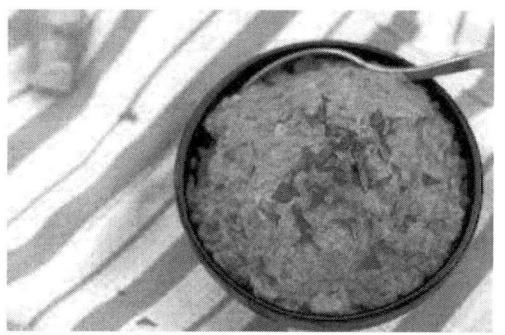

INGREDIENTS:

- 2 medium carrots, peeled and sliced
- ¼ cup butter
- ¼ cup 1% low-fat almond milk
- 2 garlic cloves

DIRECTIONS:

1. Double-boil or soak the carrots to reduce potassium if you are on a low potassium diet.
2. Boil carrots and garlic until soft. Drain.
3. Beat the carrots and garlic with butter and almond milk until smooth.

Nutrition: Calories: 168 Carbohydrate : 29g Protein: 5g Sodium: 59 Potassium: 161g Phosphorous: 57mg

167. Double-Boiled Country Style Fried Carrots

Preparation Time: 20 minutes
Cooking Time: 20 minutes
Servings: 2

INGREDIENTS:

- ½ cup canola oil
- ¼ teaspoon ground cumin
- ¼ teaspoon paprika
- ¼ teaspoon white pepper
- 3 tablespoons ketchup
- 2 cups carrots

DIRECTIONS:

1. Soak or double boil the carrots if you are on a low potassium diet.
2. Heat oil over medium heat in a skillet.
3. Fry the carrots for around 10 minutes until golden brown.
4. Drain carrots, then sprinkle with cumin, pepper, and paprika.
5. Serve with ketchup or mayo.

Nutrition: Calories: 156 Fat: 0.1g Carbohydrate: 21g Protein: 2g Sodium: 3mg Potassium: 296mg Phosphorous: 34mg

168. Broccoli-Onion Latkes

Preparation Time: 15 minutes
Cooking Time: 20 minutes
Servings: 2

INGREDIENTS:

- 3 cups broccoli florets, diced
- ½ cup onion, chopped
- 2 large eggs, beaten
- 2 tablespoons all-purpose white flour
- 2 tablespoons olive oil

DIRECTIONS:

1. Cook the broccoli for around 5 minutes until tender. Drain.
2. Mix the flour into the eggs.
3. Combine the onion, broccoli, and egg mixture and stir through.
4. Prepare olive oil in a skillet on medium-high heat.
5. Drop a spoon of the mixture onto the pan to make 4 latkes.
6. Cook each side until golden brown.
7. Drain on a paper towel and serve.

Nutrition: Calories: 140 Carbohydrate: 7g Protein: 6g Sodium: 58mg Potassium: 276mg Phosphorous: 101mg

169. Glazed Snap Peas

Preparation Time: 10 minutes
Cooking Time: 5 minutes
Servings: 2

INGREDIENTS:

- 1 cup snap peas
- 2 teaspoon Erythritol
- 1 teaspoon butter, melted
- ¾ teaspoon ground nutmeg
- ¼ teaspoon salt
- 1 cup water for cooking

DIRECTIONS:

1. Pour water into the pan. Add snap peas and bring them to a boil.
2. Boil the snap peas for 5 minutes over medium heat.
3. Then drain water and chill the snap peas.
4. Meanwhile, whisk together ground nutmeg, melted butter, salt, and Erythritol.
5. Preheat the mixture in the microwave oven for 5 seconds.
6. Pour the sweet butter liquid over the snap peas and shake them well.
7. The side dish should be served only warm.

Nutrition: Calories: 80 Fat: 2.5 Fiber: 3.9 Carbohydrate: 10.9 Protein: 4g Phosphorous: 156mg, Potassium: 225mg Sodium: 141 mg

170. Steamed Collard Greens

Preparation Time: 10 minutes
Cooking Time: 5 minutes
Servings: 2

INGREDIENTS:

- 2 cups Collard Greens
- 1 tablespoon lime juice
- 1 teaspoon olive oil
- 1 teaspoon sesame seeds
- ½ teaspoon chili flakes
- 1 cup water, for the steamer

DIRECTIONS:

1. Chop collard greens roughly.
2. Pour water in the steamer and insert rack.
3. Place the steamer bowl, add collard greens, and close the lid.
4. Steam the greens for 5 minutes.
5. After this, transfer the steamed collard greens to the salad bowl.
6. Sprinkle it with lime juice, olive oil, sesame seeds, and chili flakes.
7. Mix up greens with the help of 2 forks and leave to rest for 10 minutes before serving.

Nutrition: Calories: 43 Fat: 3.4 Fiber: 1.7 Carbohydrate: 3.4 Protein: 1.3g Phosphorous: 65mg Potassium: 67mg Sodium: 21 mg

171. Cauliflower Rice

Preparation Time: 5 minutes
Cooking Time: 10 minutes
Servings: 2

INGREDIENTS:

- 1 small head cauliflower cut into florets
- 1 tablespoon butter
- ¼ teaspoon black pepper
- ¼ teaspoon garlic powder
- ¼ teaspoon salt-free herb seasoning blend

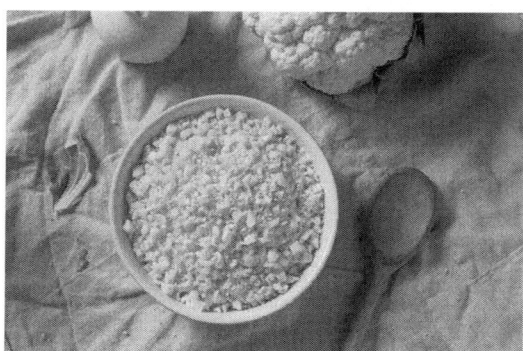

DIRECTIONS:

1. Blitz cauliflower pieces in a food processor until it has a grain-like consistency.
2. Melt butter in a saucepan and add spices.
3. Add the cauliflower rice grains and cook over low-medium heat for approximately 10 minutes.
4. Use a fork to fluff the rice before serving.
5. Serve as an alternative to rice with curries, stews, and starch to accompany meat and fish dishes.

Nutrition: Calories: 47 Carbohydrate: 4g Protein: 1g Sodium: 300mg Potassium: 206mg Phosphorous: 31mg

172. Baked Eggplants Slices

Preparation Time: 15 minutes
Cooking Time: 15 minutes
Servings: 2

INGREDIENTS:

- 1 large eggplant, trimmed

- 1 tablespoon butter, softened
- 1 teaspoon minced garlic
- 1 teaspoon salt

DIRECTIONS:

1. Slice the eggplant season it with salt. Mix up well and leave for 10 minutes to make the vegetable "give" bitter juice.
2. After this, dry the eggplant with a paper towel.
3. In the shallow bowl, mix up together minced garlic and softened butter.
4. Brush every eggplant slice with the garlic mixture.
5. Line the baking tray with baking paper. Preheat the oven to 355F.
6. Place the sliced eggplants in the tray to make 1 layer and transfer it to the oven.
7. Bake the eggplants for 15 minutes. The cooked eggplants will be tender but not soft!

Nutrition: Calories: 81 Fat: 4.2 Fiber: 6.5 Carbohydrate: 11.1g Protein: 1.9g Phosphorous: 61mg Potassium: 12mg Sodium: 5 mg

173. Fast Cabbage Cakes

Preparation Time: 15 minutes
Cooking Time: 10 minutes
Servings: 2

INGREDIENTS:

- 1 cup cauliflower, shredded
- 1 egg, beaten
- 1 teaspoon salt
- 1 teaspoon ground black pepper
- 2 tablespoons almond flour
- 1 teaspoon olive oil

DIRECTIONS:

1. Blend the shredded cabbage in the blender until you get cabbage rice.
2. Then, mix cabbage rice with the egg, salt, ground black pepper, and almond flour.
3. Pour olive oil into the skillet and preheat it.
4. Then make the small cakes with the help of 2 spoons and place them in the hot oil.
5. Roast the cabbage cakes for 4 minutes from each side over medium-low heat.

Nutrition: Calories: 227 Fat: 18.6 Fiber: 4.5 Carbohydrate: 9.5g Protein: 9.9g Phosphorous: 146mg Potassium: 217mg Sodium: 101 mg

174. Cilantro Chili Burgers

Preparation Time: 10 minutes
Cooking Time: 15 minutes
Servings: 2

INGREDIENTS:

- 1 cup red cabbage
- 3 tablespoons almond flour
- 1 tablespoon cream cheese
- 1 oz. scallions, chopped
- ½ teaspoon salt
- ½ teaspoon chili powder
- ½ cup fresh cilantro

DIRECTIONS:

1. Chop red cabbage roughly and transfer it to the blender.
2. Add fresh cilantro and blend the mixture until very smooth.

3. After this, transfer it to the bowl.
4. Add cream cheese, scallions, salt, chili powder, and almond flour.
5. Stir the mixture well.
6. Make 3 big burgers from the cabbage mixture or 6 small burgers.
7. Line the baking tray with baking paper.
8. Place the burgers in the tray.
9. Bake the cilantro burgers for 15 minutes at 360°F.
10. Flip the burgers onto another side after 8 minutes of cooking.

Nutrition:Calories: 182 Fat: 15.3 Fiber: 4.1 Carbohydrate: 8.5 Protein: 6.8 Phosphorous: 116mg Potassium: 137mg Sodium: 160mg

Smoothies & Drinks

175. Very Berry Smoothie

Preparation Time: 3 minutes
Cooking Time: 5 minutes
Servings: 2

INGREDIENTS:

- 2 quarts water
- 2 cups pomegranate seeds
- 1 cup blackberries
- 1 cup blueberries

DIRECTIONS:

1. Mix all the Ingredients in a blender.
2. Puree until smooth and creamy.
3. Transfer to a serving glass and enjoy.

Nutrition: Calories: 464 Carbohydrate: 111g Protein: 8g Fats: 4g Phosphorus: 132mg Potassium: 843mg Sodium: 16mg

176. Raspberry Peach Breakfast Smoothie

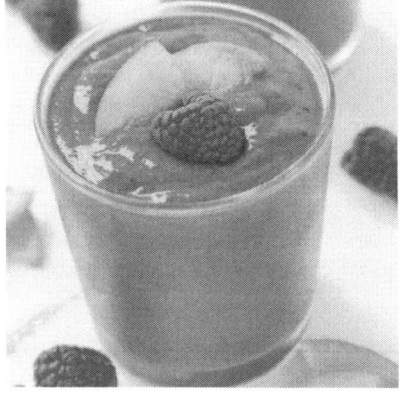

Preparation time: 5 minutes
Cooking time: 1 minute
Servings: 2

INGREDIENTS:

- 1/3 cup of raspberries, (it can be frozen)
- 1/2 peach, skin and pit removed
- 1 tablespoon of honey
- 1 cup of coconut water

DIRECTIONS:

1. Mix all ingredients together and blend it until smooth.
2. Pour and serve chilled in a tall glass or mason jar.

Nutrition: Calories: 86.3 kcal Carbohydrate: 20.6 g Protein: 1.4 g Sodium: 3 mg Potassium: 109 mg Phosphorus: 36.08 mg Dietary fiber: 2.6 g Fat: 0.31 g

177. Mango Lassi Smoothie

Preparation time: 5 minutes
Cooking time: 0 minute
Servings: 2

INGREDIENTS:

- ½ cup of plain yogurt
- ½ cup of plain water
- ½ cup of sliced mango
- 1 tablespoon of sugar
- ¼ teaspoon of cardamom
- ¼ teaspoon cinnamon
- ¼ cup lime juice

DIRECTIONS:

1. Pulse all the above ingredients in a blender until smooth (around 1 minute).

2. Pour into tall glasses or mason jars and serve chilled immediately.

Nutrition: Calories: 89.02 kcal Carbohydrate: 14.31 g Protein: 2.54 g Sodium: 30 mg Potassium: 185.67 mg Phosphorus: 67.88 mg Dietary fiber: 0.77 g Fat: 2.05 g

178. Breakfast Smoothie

Preparation Time: 15 minutes
Cooking Time: 0 minute
Servings: 2

INGREDIENTS:

- 1 cup frozen blueberries
- ½ cup pineapple chunks
- ½ cup English cucumber
- ½ apple
- ½ cup water

DIRECTIONS:

1. Put the pineapple, blueberries, cucumber, apple, and water in a blender and blend until thick and smooth.
2. Pour into 2 glasses and serve.

Nutrition: Calories: 87 Fat: 2.8 g Carbohydrate: 22g Phosphorus: 28mg Potassium: 192mg Sodium: 3mg Protein: 0.7g

179. Apple And Beet Juice Mix

Preparation time: 5 minutes
Cooking time: 5 minutes
Serving: 2

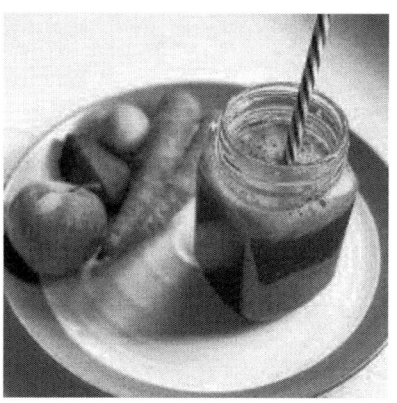

INGREDIENTS:

- ½ medium beet
- ½ medium apple
- 1 celery stalk
- 1 medium fresh carrot
- ¼ cup parsley

DIRECTIONS:

1. Juice all ingredients.
2. Pour the mixture into 2 glasses.

Nutrition: Calories: 53 Fat: 0 g Carbohydrates: 13 g Protein: 1g Phosphorus: 30 mg Potassium: 277 mg Sodium: 48 mg

180. Assorted Fresh Fruit Juice

Preparation time: 5 minutes
Cooking time: 0 minutes
Serving: 2

INGREDIENTS:

- 1 roughly chopped apple
- ¼ cup halved frozen grapes
- 1 cup ice shavings

DIRECTIONS:

1. Add all ingredients into the blender.
2. Process until smooth.
3. Pour equal portions into glasses. Serve immediately.

Nutrition: Calories: 112 Protein: 1.16g Potassium: 367 mg Sodium: 3 mg Fat: 0.5g Carbohydrate: 25.8g Phosphorus: 17.4mg

181. Berry Mint Water

Preparation time: 3 minutes
Cooking time: 5 minutes
Serving: 2

INGREDIENTS:

- 3 mint springs
- 1/2 cup blackberries
- 1/2 cup strawberries
- 8 cups water

DIRECTIONS:

1. Mix everything in a glass pitcher and allow to chill for an hour before serving.
2. Serve and enjoy!

Nutrition: Calories: 7 Protein: 0 g Sodium: 0 mg Potassium: 28 mg Phosphorus: 4 mg

182. Fennel Digestive Cooler

Preparation time: 3 minutes
Cooking time: 5 minutes
Serving: 2

INGREDIENTS:

- 1 teaspoon honey
- 1/4 teaspoon ground cloves
- 1/4 cup ground fennel seeds
- 2 cups unsweetened rice milk

DIRECTIONS:

1. Blend everything in a blender and allow to rest for 30 minutes.
2. Pour through a wire sieve lined with cheesecloth.
3. Pour into 2 glasses. Serve and enjoy!

Nutrition: Calories: 163 Protein: 3 g Sodium: 141 mg Potassium: 205 mg Phosphorus: 57 mg

183. Tropical Juice

Preparation time: 3 minutes
Cooking time: 0 minutes
Serving: 2

INGREDIENTS:

- 1 cup water
- 1/2 cup low fat coconut milk
- 1/2 cup chunked pineapple

DIRECTIONS:

1. Combine everything in a blender.
2. Blend until smooth.
3. Pour into 2 glasses. Serve and enjoy!

Nutrition: Calories: 55 Protein: 7 g Sodium: 111 mg Potassium: 129 mg Phosphorus: 11 mg

184. Green Tea with Arugula Leaves, Lime, And Kale Leaves

Preparation time: 5 minutes
Cooking time: 5 minutes
Serving: 2

INGREDIENTS:

- 1 quart (4 cups) filtered or spring water
- 4 tea bags green tea
- 2 pieces, large lime, sliced into bite-sized wedges, remove pips
- ¼ cup, tightly packed arugula leaves, rinsed well, drained
- ¼ cup, tightly packed kale leaves, rinsed well, drained

DIRECTIONS:

1. Place all ingredients into a large pitcher. Mix while gently bruising lime wedges and leaves. Set aside for at least 4 to 6 hours in the fridge.
2. Strain out leaves and tea bags. Pour green tea with lime wedges. Always serve chilled.

Nutrition: Protein: 0.47g Potassium: 60 mg Sodium: 12 mg

185. Winter Berry Milkshake

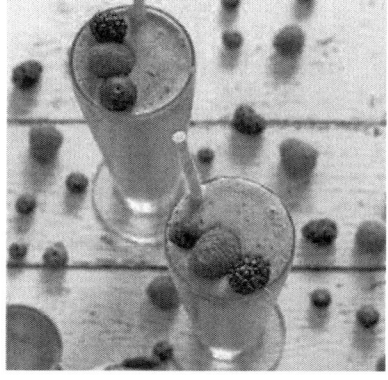

Preparation time: 3 minutes
Cooking time: 5 minutes
Serving: 2
INGREDIENTS:

- 3 ice cubes
- 1/2 cup blackberries
- 1/2 cup blueberries
- 1 cup unsweetened rice milk

DIRECTIONS:

1. Combine everything in a blender.
2. Blend until smooth.
3. Pour into 4 glasses. Serve and enjoy!

Nutrition: Calories: 45 Protein: 2 g Sodium: 29 mg Potassium: 118 mg Phosphorus: 33 mg

186. Pineapple Juice

Preparation Time: 5 minutes
Cooking Time: 0 minutes
Servings: 2
INGREDIENTS:

- ½ cup canned pineapple
- 1 cup water

DIRECTIONS:

1. Blend all ingredients and serve over ice.

Nutrition: Calories: 135 Protein: 0 g Carbohydrate: 0 g Fat: 0 g Sodium: 0 mg Potassium: 180 mg Phosphorus: 8 mg

Desserts

187. Pudding Glass with Banana and Whipped Cream

Preparation Time: 15 minutes

Cooking Time: 0 minutes

Servings: 2

INGREDIENTS:

- 2 portions of banana cream pudding mix
- 2 1/2 cups rice milk
- 8 oz. dairy whipped cream
- 12 oz. vanilla wafers

DIRECTIONS:

1. Put vanilla wafers in a pan and, in another bowl, mix banana cream pudding and rice milk. Boil the ingredients while blending them slowly.
2. Pour the mixture over the wafers and make 2 or 3 layers. Put the pan in the fridge for one hour and afterward spread the whipped topping over the dessert.
3. Put it back in the refrigerator within 2 hours and serve it cold in transparent glasses. Serve and enjoy!

Nutrition: Calories: 255 Protein: 3 g Carbohydrate: 19g Fat: 3g Sodium: 275 mg Potassium: 50 mg Phosphorus: 40 mg

188. Pumpkin Cheesecake

Preparation Time: 15 minutes

Cooking Time: 55 minutes

Servings: 2

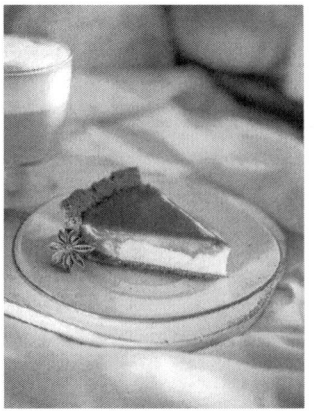

INGREDIENTS:

- 1 egg white
- 1 wafer crumb, 9-inch pie crust
- 1/2 small bowl of granular sugar
- 1 teaspoon vanilla extract
- 1 teaspoon pumpkin pie flavoring
- 1/2 bowl pumpkin cream
- 1/2 small bowl liquid egg substitute
- 8 tablespoons frozen topping, for desserts
- 16 oz. cream cheese

DIRECTIONS:

1. Brush pie crust with egg white and cook for 5 minutes in a preheated oven from 375°F from 375°F now down to 350°F.
2. Put sugar, vanilla, and cream cheese, beating with a mixer in a large cup until smooth. Beat the egg substitute and add pumpkin cream with pie flavoring: blend everything until softened.
3. Put the pumpkin mixture in a pie shell and bake for 50 minutes to set the center. Then let the pie cool down and

then put it in the fridge. When you wish to, serve it in 8 slices, putting some topping on it. Serve and enjoy!

Nutrition: Calories: 364 Protein: 5 g Carbohydrate: 23g Fat: 2g Sodium: 245 mg Potassium: 125 mg Phosphorus: 65 mg

189. Small Chocolate Cakes

Preparation Time: 15 minutes
Cooking Time: 1 minute
Servings: 2

INGREDIENTS:

1. 1 box of angel food cake mix
2. 1 box lemon cake mix
3. water
4. nonstick cooking spray or batter
5. dark chocolate small squared chops and chocolate powder

DIRECTIONS:

1. Use a transparent kitchen cooking bag and put inside both lemon cake mixes, angel food mix, and chocolate squared chops. Mix everything and put water to prepare a small cupcake.
2. Put the mix in a mold to prepare a cupcake containing the ingredients and put in microwave for a one-minute-high temperature.
3. Slip the cupcake out of the mold, put it on a dish, let it cool, and put some more chocolate crumbs on it. Serve and enjoy!

Nutrition: Calories: 95 Carbohydrate: 28g Fat: 3g Protein: 1 g Sodium: 162 mg Potassium: 15 mg Phosphorus: 80 mg

190. Amarena Dessert

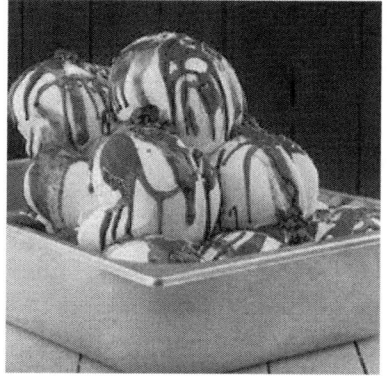

Preparation Time: 5 minutes
Cooking Time: 30 minutes
Servings: 2

INGREDIENTS:

- 3.5 oz. mascarpone
- 1.7 oz. sour cream
- 1 packet of vanilla sugar
- 1.7 oz. Amarena cherries with juice
- 1 tablespoon lime juice
- some grated lime zests
- 4 ladyfingers

DIRECTIONS:

1. Mix the mascarpone with sour cream, vanilla sugar, lime juice, and zest until creamy. Break the sponge fingers and place them in two dessert bowls. Pour half of the Amarena cherries on top and pour in the cream mixture. Place the remaining Amarena cherries on top.

Nutrition: Calories: 360kcal Protein: 3 Fat: 25g Carbohydrates: 31g Potassium: 132mg Phosphate: 85mg

191. Strawberry Ice Cream

Preparation time: 5 minutes
Cooking time: 5 minutes

Servings: 2

INGREDIENTS:

- ½ cup Stevia
- 1 tablespoon Lemon juice
- ¾ cup non-dairy coffee creamer
- 10 oz. strawberries
- 1 cup crushed ice

DIRECTIONS:

1. Blend everything in a blend until smooth.
2. Freeze until frozen.
3. Serve.

Nutrition: Calories: 94.4 Fat: 6g Carbohydrate: 8.3g Phosphorus: 25mg Potassium: 108mg Sodium: 25mg Protein: 1.3g

192. Grilled Peach Sundaes

Preparation Time: 15 minutes
Cooking Time: 5 minutes
Servings: 2

INGREDIENTS:

- 1 tablespoon toasted unsweetened coconut
- 1 teaspoon canola oil
- 2 peaches, halved and pitted
- 2 scoops non-fat vanilla yogurt, frozen

DIRECTIONS:

1. Brush the peaches with oil and grill until tender.
2. Place peach halves on a bowl and top with frozen yogurt and coconut.

Nutrition: Calories: 61; carbs: 2g; protein: 2g; fats: 6g; phosphorus: 32mg; potassium: 85mg; sodium: 30mg

193. Almond Butter Mousse

Preparation Time: 7 minutes
Cooking Time: 7 minutes
Servings: 2

INGREDIENTS:

- 2 strawberries
- 1 cup of coconut milk
- 1/2 teaspoon vanilla extract
- 2 teaspoon Erythritol
- 4 tablespoons almond butter
- ¾ teaspoon ground cinnamon

DIRECTIONS:

1. Pour coconut milk in the food processor.
2. Add vanilla extract, Erythritol, almond butter, and ground cinnamon.
3. Blend the mixture until smooth.
4. Ten transfer it in the saucepan and start to preheat it over the medium heat.
5. Stir it all the time.
6. When the mousse starts to be thick, remove it from the heat and stir.
7. Pour the mousse into the serving glasses.
8. Slice the strawberries.
9. Top the mousse with the strawberries.

Nutrition: Calories: 321 Fat: 31.1 Fiber: 4.4 Carbohydrate: 9.6 Protein: 6.4

194. Keto Panna Cotta

Preparation Time: 10 minutes
Cooking Time: 10 minutes
Servings: 2

INGREDIENTS:

- 1 cup heavy cream
- 1 teaspoon vanilla extract
- 2 teaspoons Erythritol
- 2 teaspoon blackberries
- 1 tablespoon gelatin powder
- 5 tablespoons water

DIRECTIONS:

1. Pour heavy cream in the saucepan and bring it to boil.
2. Meanwhile, mix up together water with gelatin powder. Let gelatin powder to soak water.
3. When the heavy cream is boiling, remove it from the heat, add vanilla extract.
4. Chill the heavy cream to the 104F.
5. Mash the blackberries with Erythritol.
6. Mix up together soaked gelatin and chilled heavy cream. When the mixture is smooth pour it into the pannacotta glasses.
7. Chill the mixture in the fridge for 20 minutes.
8. After this, top Pannacotta with the mashed blackberries.
9. Chill the dessert in the fridge until it is solid (appx.20 minutes).

Nutrition: Calories: 226 Fat: 22.2 Fiber: 0.2 Carbohydrate: 2.2 Protein: 4.3 Phosphorus: 39 mg Potassium: 54 mg Sodium: 31 mg

195. Spiced Peaches

Preparation time: 5 minutes
Cooking time: 10 minutes
Servings: 2
INGREDIENTS:

- 1 cup canned peaches with juices
- ½ teaspoon cornstarch
- 1 teaspoon ground cloves
- 1 teaspoon ground cinnamon
- 1 teaspoon ground nutmeg
- ½ lemon zest
- ½ cup water

DIRECTIONS:

1. Drain peaches.
2. Combine cinnamon, cornstarch, nutmeg, ground cloves, and lemon zest in a pan on the stove.
3. Heat on medium heat and add peaches.
4. Bring to a boil, reduce the heat and simmer for 10 minutes.
5. Serve.

Nutrition: Calories: 70 Fat: 0g Carbohydrate: 14g Phosphorus: 23mg Potassium: 176mg Sodium: 3mg Protein: 1g

196. Pumpkin Cheesecake Bar

Preparation time: 10 minutes
Cooking time: 50 minutes
Servings: 2
INGREDIENTS:

- 2 ½ tablespoons unsalted butter
- 4 ounces cream cheese
- ½ cup all-purpose white flour
- 3 tablespoons golden brown sugar
- ¼ cup granulated sugar
- ½ cup pureed pumpkin
- 2 egg whites
- 1 teaspoon ground cinnamon
- 1 teaspoon ground nutmeg
- 1 teaspoon vanilla extract

DIRECTIONS:

1. Preheat the oven to 350ºF.
2. Mix flour and brown sugar in a bowl.
3. Mix in the butter to form 'breadcrumbs.
4. Place ¾ of this mixture in a dish.
5. Bake in the oven for 15 minutes. Remove and cool.
6. Lightly whisk the egg and fold in the cream cheese, sugar, pumpkin, cinnamon, nutmeg, and vanilla until smooth.
7. Pour this mixture over the oven-baked base and sprinkle with the rest of the breadcrumbs from earlier.
8. Bake in the oven for 30 to 35 minutes more.
9. Cool, slice, and serve.

Nutrition: Calories: 248 Fat: 13g Carbohydrate: 33g Phosphorus: 67mg Potassium: 96mg Sodium: 146mg Protein: 4g

197. Blueberry Mini Muffins

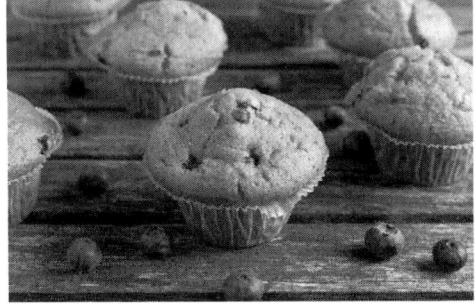

Preparation time: 10 minutes
Cooking time: 35 minutes
Servings: 2

INGREDIENTS:

- 3 egg whites
- ¼ cup all-purpose white flour
- 1 tablespoon coconut flour
- 1 teaspoon baking soda
- 1 teaspoon grated nutmeg
- 1 teaspoon vanilla extract
- 1 teaspoon stevia
- ¼ cup fresh blueberries

DIRECTIONS:

1. Preheat the oven to 325ºF.
2. Mix all the ingredients in a bowl.
3. Divide the batter into 4 and spoon into a lightly oiled muffin tin.
4. Bake in the oven for 15 to 20 minutes or until it is well cooked.
5. Cool and serve.

Nutrition: Calories: 62 Fat: 0g Carbohydrate: 9g Phosphorus: 103mg Potassium: 65mg Sodium: 62mg Protein: 4g

198. Lemon Mousse

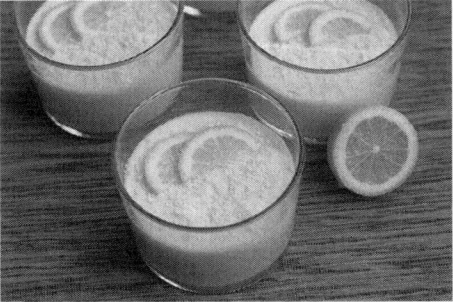

Preparation time: 10 + chill time
Cooking time: 10 minutes
Servings: 2

INGREDIENTS:

- 1 cup coconut cream
- 8 ounces cream cheese, soft
- ¼ cup fresh lemon juice
- 3 pinches salt
- 1 teaspoon lemon liquid stevia

DIRECTIONS:

1. Preheat your oven to 350°F.
2. Grease a ramekin with butter.
3. Beat cream, cream cheese, fresh lemon juice, salt, and lemon liquid stevia in a mixer.
4. Pour batter into a ramekin.
5. Bake for 10 minutes, then transfer the mousse to a serving glass.
6. Let it chill for 2 hours and serve.
7. Enjoy!

Nutrition: Calories: 395 Fat: 31g Carbohydrates: 3g Protein: 5g Potassium: 51 mg Sodium: 50 mg Phosphorus: 252 mg

199. Raspberry Popsicle

Preparation Time: 2 hours
Cooking Time: 15 minutes
Servings: 2

INGREDIENTS:

- 1 ½ cups raspberries
- 2 cups of water

DIRECTIONS:

1. Take a pan and fill it up with water
2. Add raspberries
3. Place it over medium heat and bring to water to a boil
4. Reduce the heat and simmer for 15 minutes
5. Remove heat and pour the mix into Popsicle molds
6. Add a popsicle stick and let it chill for 2 hours
7. Serve and enjoy!

Nutrition: Calories: 58 Fat: 0.4g Carbohydrates: 0g Protein: 1.4g Phosphorus: 17 mg Potassium: 180 mg Sodium: 11 mg

200. Coconut Loaf

Preparation Time: 15 minutes
Cooking Time: 40 minutes
Servings: 4

INGREDIENTS:

- 1 ½ tablespoons coconut flour
- ¼ teaspoon baking powder
- 1/8 teaspoon salt
- 1 tablespoon coconut oil, melted
- 1 whole egg

DIRECTIONS:

1. Preheat your oven to 350°F
2. Add coconut flour, baking powder, salt
3. Add coconut oil, eggs and stir well until mixed
4. Leave the batter for several minutes
5. Pour half the batter onto the baking pan
6. Spread it to form a circle, repeat with remaining batter
7. Bake in the oven for 10 minutes
8. Once a golden-brown texture comes, let it cool and serve
9. Enjoy!

Nutrition: Calories: 297 Fat: 14g Carbohydrates: 15g Protein: 15g Potassium: 72 mg Sodium: 19 mg Phosphorus: 24 mg

201. Dessert Cocktail

Preparation time: 1 minute

Cooking time: 0 minute

Servings: 2

INGREDIENTS:

- 1 cup cranberry juice
- 1 cup fresh ripe strawberries, washed and hull removed
- 2 tablespoon lime juice
- ¼ cup white sugar
- 8 ice cubes

DIRECTIONS:

1. Combine all the ingredients in a blender until smooth and creamy.
2. Pour the liquid into tall and chilled glasses and serve cold.

Nutrition: Calories: 92 Carbohydrate: 23.5g Protein: 0.5g Sodium: 3.62mg Potassium: 103.78mg Phosphorus: 17.86mg Dietary fiber: 0.84g Fat: 0.17g

202. Baked Egg Custard

Preparation time: 15 minutes

Cooking time: 30 minutes

Servings: 2

INGREDIENTS:

- 2 medium eggs, at room temperature
- ¼ cup semi-skimmed milk
- 3 tablespoons white sugar
- ½ teaspoon nutmeg
- 1 teaspoon vanilla extract

DIRECTIONS:

1. Preheat your oven at 375ºF
2. Mix all the ingredients in a mixing bowl and beat with a hand mixer for a few seconds until creamy and uniform.
3. Pour the mixture into lightly greased muffin tins.
4. Bake for 25–30 minutes or until the knife you place inside comes out clean.

Nutrition: Calories: 96.56 Carbohydrate: 10.5g Protein: 3.5g Sodium: 37.75mg Potassium: 58.19mg Phosphorus: 58.76mg Dietary fiber: 0.06g Fat: 2.91g

Meal Plans

WEEK 1

Day	Breakfast	Lunch	Snacks	Dinner
1	Mexican Scrambled Eggs in Tortilla	Beef Ragu	Veggie Snack	Apricot Chicken Wings
2	Turkey and Spinach Scramble on Melba Toast	Cajun Catfish	Healthy Spiced Nuts	Asparagus Shrimp Linguini
3	Mexican Style Burritos	Carrot & Ginger Chicken Noodles	Roasted Asparagus	Baked Cod with Salsa
4	Buckwheat and Grapefruit Porridge	Cherry Chicken Salad	Low-Fat Mango Salsa	Baked Fennel & Garlic Sea Bass
5	Vegetable Omelet	Chicken Sauté	Vinegar & Salt Kale	Baked Fish à la Mushrooms
6	Feta Mint Omelet	Chicken Strawberry Green Lettuce Salad with Ginger-Lime Dressing	Carrot and Parsnips French Fries	Beef Brochettes
7	Pumpkin Apple Muffins	Chicken Strawberry Spinach Salad with Ginger-Lime Dressing	Apple & Strawberry Snack	Beef Pot Roast

WEEK 2

Day	Breakfast	Lunch	Snacks	Dinner
1	Feta And Bell Pepper Quiche	Chinese Beef Wraps	Candied Macadamia Nuts	Creamy Chicken
2	Quinoa Porridge	Cilantro and Chili Infused Swordfish	Popcorn with Sugar and Spice	Creamy Turkey
3	Egg and Veggie Muffins	Cilantro Drumsticks	Baba Ghanouj	Fruity Chicken Salad
4	Berry Chia with Yogurt	Cilantro-Lime Flounder	Herbal Cream Cheese Tartines	Ginger & Bean Sprout Steak Stir-Fry
5	Arugula Eggs with Chili Peppers	Citrus Tuna Ceviche	Mixes of Snacks	Glazed Salmon
6	Eggplant Chicken Sandwich	Cooked Tilapia with Mango Salsa	Spicy Crab Dip	Grilled Chicken Pizza
7	Grandma's Pancake Special	Country Fried Steak	Blueberry-Ricotta Swirl	Haddock & Buttered Leeks

WEEK 3

Day	Breakfast	Lunch	Snacks	Dinner
1	Raspberry Peach Breakfast Smoothie	Halibut with Lemon Caper Sauce	Carrot and Parsnips French Fries	Spanish Cod in Sauce
2	Fast Microwave Egg Scramble	Herb-Crusted Baked Haddock	Apple & Strawberry Snack	Spiced Lamb Burgers
3	Summer Veggie Omelet	Homemade Burgers	Candied Macadamia Nuts	Sweet Glazed Salmon
4	Apple and Onion Omelet	Jambalaya	Popcorn with Sugar and Spice	Thai Spiced Halibut
5	Avocado Toast with Egg	Lamb with Prunes	Baba Ghanouj	Tuna Casserole
6	Breakfast Burrito	Lamb with Zucchini & Couscous	Herbal Cream Cheese Tartines	Tuna Noodle Casserole
7	Mushroom and Red Pepper Omelet	Lemon & Herb Chicken Wraps	Mixes of Snacks	Turkey Sausages

WEEK 4

Day	Breakfast	Lunch	Snacks	Dinner
1	Avocado Toast with Egg	Salmon & Pesto Salad	Easy No-Bake Coconut Cookies	Parmesan And Basil Turkey Salad
2	Breakfast Burrito	Sardine Fish Cakes	Roasted Chili-Vinegar Peanuts	Poached Gennaro/Seabass with Red Peppers
3	Mushroom and Red Pepper Omelet	Shrimp and Asparagus Linguine	Veggie Snack	Pork Loins with Leeks
4	Mexican Scrambled Eggs in Tortilla	Shrimp Paella	Healthy Spiced Nuts	Pork with Bell Pepper
5	Turkey and Spinach Scramble on Melba Toast	Shrimp Scampi Linguine	Roasted Asparagus	Red and Green Grapes Chicken Salad with Curry
6	Mexican Style Burritos	Shrimp Szechuan	Low-Fat Mango Salsa	Roast Beef
7	Buckwheat and Grapefruit Porridge	Southern Fried Chicken	Vinegar & Salt Kale	Rosemary Chicken

Conclusion

I hope you will have a better grasp of Renal Diet after reading this book than you had before. I am sure that with all these information you will start following Renal Diet easily.

The first reason for following this diet is that Renal Diet is more effective in reducing blood pressure. According to the medical journal, if you want to reduce blood pressure using a specific diet then renal diet has the highest possibility to be effective than other diets.

Moreover, Renal Diet also has a wide range of advantages to our health. Here are some noticeable advantages that I believe would be nice to know.

Renal diet could be helpful in reducing cholesterol levels as well as triglyceride. In fact, it is also effective in reducing LDL levels. One of the reasons why persons with cardiovascular disease should eat a Renal Diet is because of this.

Renal diet is also beneficial for muscle strength. Meats like beef and fish are high in protein which makes them an important food to boost muscle strength. Furthermore, Renal Diet also contains low levels of fructose which could help in muscle repair and recovery.

Another advantage is that Renal Diet also contains many vitamins and minerals. Aside from carbs, renal diet also includes some high-quality proteins like eggs and fish which are rich in B vitamins. This will enhance the working of our brain and keep the memory active.

Renal Diet has low levels of saturated fats as well as trans fat. Moreover, it contains high levels of fiber. Fibers reduce cholesterol absorption therefore we can have a lower chance for having high levels of cholesterol in our body.

It's also important to understand that the goal of this diet is not only to reduce waste products, but also to increase overall health. To do this, your body needs to get the nutrients it needs and the energy that it requires. "It's not enough to know how much food and how much calories you're eating; you need to know what kind of calories you're eating. Diets that only restrict protein and calories tend to cause problems in other body systems."

The diet is simple and can be carried out in most foods. It rarely requires supplements or specific food choices.

Renal Diet together with some exercise will help you to change your lifestyle in a better way, improving your health and preventing or helping you to live with CKD.

Made in the USA
Monee, IL
12 September 2022

13811949R00077